The Alzheimer's Answer

The Alzheimer's Answer

Reduce Your Risk and Keep Your Brain Healthy

MARWAN NOEL SABBAGH, MD

Director, the Cleo Roberts Center for Clinical Research
Sun Health Research Institute

WILEY

John Wiley & Sons, Inc.

Published by John Wiley & Sons, Inc., Hoboken, New Jersey
Published simultaneously in Canada

Illustration credits: pages 36, 37, 39, 246, courtesy of the NIA, www.nia.nih.gov/Alzheimers/ Resources; pages 38, 41 (top), provided by Dr. Thomas Beach of Sun Health Research Institute; page 41 (bottom), provided by Athena diagnostics with permission; page 51, courtesy of the NIA 2004–2005 Alzheimer's disease progress report; pages 100, 102, Drs. Alex Roher and Thomas Beach of Sun Health Research Institute.

The Alzheimer's Questionnaire on page 239 is courtesy of the Sun Health Research Institute.

Design and composition by Navta Associates, Inc.

The information contained in this book is not intended to serve as a replacement for professional medical advice. Any use of the information in this book is at the reader's discretion. The author and the publisher specifically disclaim any and all liability arising directly or indirectly from the use or application of any information contained in this book. A health care professional should be consulted regarding your specific situation.

For general information about our other products and services, please contact our Customer Care Department within the United States at (800) 762–2974, outside the United States at (317) 572–3993 or fax (317) 572–4002.

Wiley also publishes its books in a variety of electronic formats. Some content that appears in print may not be available in electronic books. For more information about Wiley products, visit our web site at www.wiley.com.

Library of Congress Cataloging-in-Publication Data:

Sabbagh, Marwan Noel.
  The Alzheimer's answer : reduce your risk and keep your brain healthy / Marwan Noel Sabbagh ; foreword by Justice Sandra Day O'Connor.
      p. cm.
  Includes bibliographical references and index.
  ISBN 978-0-470-04494-0 (cloth)
  1. Alzheimer's disease--Prevention--Popular works. 2. Self-care, Health--Popular works. I. Title.
  RC523.2.S23 2008
  616.8'3105--dc22   2007044823

Printed in the United States of America

10 9 8 7 6 5 4 3 2

To my beloved wife, Ida, who inspires me.

Contents

Foreword by
Justice Sandra Day O'Connor

Alzheimer's has become a word that most people know—and fear. Some project that 40 percent or more of people over eighty will have Alzheimer's disease. A high percentage of families have a member afflicted with the disease and have experienced the long, slow process of mental and physical deterioration that comes with it. Such families also experience the stress and problems of the caregivers of people with the disease. To watch the slow debilitation of a person you love is nothing less than devastating.

Alzheimer's was not well known or recognized before 1980. It was first identified by Dr. Alois Alzheimer. Many cases of so-called senility or dementia were no doubt Alzheimer's but were not then known as such. Today, Alzheimer's is a household word.

As a spouse, child, relative, or friend of a person afflicted with Alzheimer's, one naturally asks, "What causes the disease?" "What can be done to treat it?" "What can be done to prevent it from occurring?" and "What can I do?"

There are a number of books and articles about Alzheimer's already in circulation. I am the wife of a beloved husband who suffers from the disease. I read all that I can on the subject. This book, *The Alzheimer's Answer,* has succinctly and clearly addressed and answered my questions. And it has given me some hope that my children can live their lives in a way that may enable them to avoid developing the disease. There are actions each of us can take and lifestyles that will enable us to prevent the possible onset of

Alzheimer's, despite some negative and unavoidable risk factors such as age, gender, and genetic history.

In this clearly written and well-organized volume, one can discover what medical information to request, what diet to follow, and what weight level to attain in order to reduce the risk. Dr. Sabbagh has provided a much needed and extremely useful book about a much dreaded disease.

Acknowledgments

There are many who have supported and assisted me with this book. First, I would like to thank my agent, Jodie Rhodes, who made things happen. Second, I would like to thank Paul Simpson, PhD, who put me on the right path. I would like to acknowledge the efforts of Kate Petersen for her writing assistance in the preparation of this book. Her efforts are gratefully appreciated.

I would like to thank my colleagues at SHRI. This includes Drs. Thomas Beach, Rena Li, Larry Sparks, Alex Roher, Joseph Rogers, Donald Connor, LihFen Lue, Douglas Walker, and Yong Shen. I would also like to acknowledge the physicians and scientists who, at my request, provided me with scientific literature that served as the raw material for this book. I am also grateful to colleagues from other institutions for providing me raw materials. These include Robert Green, MD, MPH, from Boston University; John Ringman, MD, from UCLA; Scott Turner, MD, PhD, from the University of Michigan; James Joseph, MD, from Tufts University; and Joseph Quinn, MD, from Oregon Health Sciences University.

I would like to thank my editor, Deborah Baker. I am grateful to Jamie Hewlett for her expert proofreading and constructive comments. I would like to thank in particular my administrative assistant, Bonnie Tigner. I wish to thank Selma Marks, Esq., and Walter Nieri, MD, both of whom facilitated the contact with Justice O'Connor.

I would also like to thank Patricia Lynch, director of communications from NIA, for providing me access to reprint some of the figures in this book.

I am grateful to my mentors over the years who have helped guide me toward a career focused on Alzheimer's disease. These include Greg Cole, PhD, of UCLA; Abdu Adem, PhD, of Karolinska Institute; Agneta Nordberg, MD, of Karolinksa Institute; Rachelle Doody, MD, PhD, of Baylor College of Medicine; and Leon Thal, MD, of UCSD. Dr. Thal recently passed away. As my greatest mentor and a giant in the field of Alzheimer's clinical research, he had the biggest impact on my career. I owe all of my success and much of my prosperity to him. I miss him greatly.

I would like to thank my family for suffering through the book with me: my wife, Ida; my children, Habib and Elias; my parents, Adib and Vivi Sabbagh; and my brother, Hadil.

Finally, I would to thank all my patients and the residents of Sun City who inspire me and helped me as much as I have helped them.

A portion of the proceeds of this book will be used to support ongoing research at the Sun Health Research Institute.

Introduction

My mother-in-law, Barbara Crocker, lived with my family for ten years before she began to show signs of dementia. I then experienced firsthand the increasing toll memory loss, delusion, "sundowning" (increased confusion as afternoon becomes evening), disorientation, and agitation takes on both a patient and a family. She was diagnosed, in time, with normal pressure hydrocephalus coupled with Alzheimer's disease. My wife, also a physician, and I agonized over what to do. We kept Barbara at home for as long as we could, enlisting a daytime caregiver during the week, who was relieved by another on the weekends. I took up the night shift. It got to the point where we could no longer care for her, and so to honor her wishes and not prolong her life through more aggressive means such as surgery or life support, we admitted her to a hospice. She passed away after a few weeks.

My close involvement with my mother-in-law during her bout with Alzheimer's gave me great compassion and empathy for the millions of caregivers, so often family members, who are placed in a similar situation, given what they face day in and day out. In addition, I share the concern of the children and siblings of patients with Alzheimer's who may worry and wonder, "Is this genetic? Am I next?" This book is written for those people, and for anyone who is concerned that he or she may face a future with Alzheimer's.

Beginning when I was a freshman in college, I wanted to study and to treat Alzheimer's disease. I believe that desire stemmed from a fear of aging. To me, Alzheimer's is the embodiment of all that is sad and destructive about growing old. So I set out on a career quest to stamp out this disease. Working in the retirement community of Sun City, Arizona, I have learned a lot about dementia and Alzheimer's disease. Now that drugs are becoming available and affordable, I prescribe medications that are intended to help patients with Alzheimer's, with the hope that their dementia will not overtake their lives; perhaps these medications will enable them to enjoy their friends, family, and activities longer. Often, I counsel families on what to expect and how to address specific issues that impact the patient and immediate relatives, such as driving, independence, supervision of medications, behavior, mood, and, later in the disease, perhaps nursing home or other placement.

I have also become much more optimistic about aging. As the clinical director of the Brain and Body Donation Program at Sun Health Research Institute, where I am responsible for regular assessments of its participants, every day I see folks who are at the oldest of the old-age spectrum, and many are in perfect mental shape. This program has been in existence for more than eighteen years and has enrolled more than 2,400 donors (more than 1 percent of the current combined populations of the surrounding retirement communities of Sun City, City West, and Sun City Grand have been or are members). All the donors have volunteered specifically for the program and are highly motivated. Of these, almost 1,000 donors have already donated their brains; these organs have been used to propel important scientific discoveries. Currently, more than 900 living donors come regularly to our center for assessments of their medical, family, medication, and health habit history, as well as physical and neurological examinations and complete cognitive assessments. All of this information is gathered into a custom-designed database that allows our clinical and scientific researchers to explore why Alzheimer's develops. A major strength of our Brain and Body Donation Program has been the large number of donors who are nondemented. These subjects serve as a control population and permit our scientists and research physicians to discover mechanisms of healthy aging and disease, and differences between normal aging and diseases such as Alzheimer's.

Indeed, I have become accustomed to seeing elderly far into their eighties and nineties and even centenarians who are cognitively well and lead active lives in spite of other health problems. In Sun City, where a resident has to be fifty-five years old to qualify to live there, we joke that you're not even old until you hit eighty.

I also give many community lectures in which I discuss ways to treat Alzheimer's and its attendant complications. Many in the audience come to see if they are getting Alzheimer's. I tell them, "If you go from your living room to your kitchen and cannot remember why you went there but you remember why a few minutes later, that is a 'senior moment.' If you go from your living room to your kitchen and cannot remember that it is your kitchen, that is *not* a senior moment, and you should see a doctor."

In the same way, if you haven't seen someone in twenty years and can't remember his or her name when you run into that person in the airport, that's a senior moment, or perhaps simply the result of this individual's appearing in a context you don't relate with him or her, just as you might not recognize your mailman if you bump into him in a swimsuit on the beach. But if you find yourself confusing the names or personalities of your children with those of your spouse, parents, or siblings, that is not okay and you should see a doctor.

At these lectures, I say that I want to work myself out of a job. I really mean that. I get up every day hoping to see a world without Alzheimer's disease. I hope this book can help toward achieving that goal. I practice what I preach in my own life and adhere to the guidelines set forth in this book.

Often people ask me, "Are there things I can do to keep from getting Alzheimer's disease?" In short, I believe there are, and in the following chapters I summarize what we know and what we don't know about dementia and ways to forestall or slow it.

Think of this as a guidebook for a fast-changing medical future: Like any good guidebook, it provides options for the journey and points out some of the well-known historical landmarks of Alzheimer's research and what to expect of the disease. But it also reveals some lesser-known aspects of Alzheimer's pathology, prevention ideas, and some detours that may help you bypass the disease altogether. These are real recommendations based on the best and most current evidence from the medical literature. My goal is to translate some of the complex scientific ideas driving Alzheimer's treatment and research today into practical information that you can use to assess your risk and develop a prevention strategy. Throughout, I've included experiences from my clinical practice to illustrate the science.

The good news is that we know a lot more about this devastating illness than most people are aware of. We understand the changes that occur in the brains of people with Alzheimer's disease and, more important, how these processes occur and what environmental factors influence them.

The timing of this book is not accidental: The first wave of the 77 million American baby boomers begins retiring in 2008. We are therefore looking harder than ever for ways to prevent this dreaded disease.

This book is divided into four parts. In the first part, we will explore what Alzheimer's is and its relationship to dementia. I'll identify some major risk factors and provide a useful set of tools for you to begin to assess your personal Alzheimer's risk. Finally, we'll explore whether preventing Alzheimer's is a reasonable goal. I argue that it is and, moreover, that prevention is sorely needed.

In the second part, each chapter will outline what we know, the scientific basis for that knowledge, and what questions are still unanswered. Based on what we do know and can reasonably infer, I will make real recommendations based on the best and most current evidence.

In the third part, I will address the treatment of Alzheimer's disease and its complications, outlining the available therapies, the advantages and downsides to each, and some other treatments that are in the offing.

Finally, in the last part of the book, I will talk about the future of Alzheimer's: where the research is headed, how fast or slow it's moving, and what the prognosis might look like in twenty or fifty years. This part includes questionnaires that will help you determine your risks for developing Alzheimer's and whether you are developing symptoms that may be worth checking out.

Keep in mind that this book focuses on Alzheimer's almost exclusively and not on other dementias. This is partially because we know a lot more about Alzheimer's than about other dementias. For the most part, the recommendations that apply to Alzheimer's have not necessarily been proven to apply to other dementias.

While this book might be reassuring or even uplifting, it is not meant to lull you into a false sense of assurance; after reading it, you will see there is still a great deal we don't know about Alzheimer's. For example, from a global perspective, most of the population-based studies have not been proven in controlled clinical trials. At Sun Health Research Institute, however, we do perform such trials precisely to eliminate the bias inherent in doing research. After all, as investigators, we often want to believe that a drug or compound really works. So during the clinical trials, we blind ourselves to the real treatment assignment by giving some participants a placebo. That way, neither the investigator nor the participant knows who is getting the real medication versus the placebo. In this manner, we take every precaution that the outcome we observe is due to good science and not to chance or to some predetermined desire for a particular outcome.

As with any rapidly changing field, what we understand about Alzheimer's today may not pan out in the future, or it may be modified by new discoveries. Nothing in this book is the final say, to be sure. In nearly every chapter there is more to be discovered about the subject, and as those discoveries are made, recommendations will no doubt change or become more specific.

Some of my medical and scientific colleagues may disagree with some of my points or recommendations, especially those not yet supported by robust clinical trial data or consensus guidelines. If you decide to incorporate any of the recommendations from this book into your medical routine, please consult your physician first.

PART I

Preventing Alzheimer's

1

Alzheimer's Disease

A lot of senior citizens in Sun City, Arizona, panic when they forget where they put their glasses or can't remember the name of someone they met at a cocktail party. Many middle-aged professionals, in the prime of their lives, worry as well. Naturally, one's first thought is Alzheimer's. How can you tell if this type of memory loss is the kind that is entirely natural and expected with age or the first sign of the onset of Alzheimer's, which is truly an illness? First, you have to know what Alzheimer's is and what it is not.

A Definition

Alzheimer's disease causes gradual memory loss, a decline in the ability to perform routine tasks, disorientation, difficulty in learning, loss of language skills, impairment of judgment, and personality changes. As the disease progresses, people with Alzheimer's become unable to care for themselves, and their loss of brain function eventually leads to the failure of other systems in the body, causing death three to twenty years from the onset of symptoms.

More simply, Alzheimer's is a brain disease. It is *not* normal aging. It affects cognitive function in multiple areas of the brain. As the life span in the United States and other industrialized nations continues to increase, Alzheimer's disease has emerged as one of the most common brain disorders. It looms large not only because it is becoming increasingly common or prevalent, but also because of its terrifying course. What begins as benign forgetfulness ends by ultimately ravaging the entire mind.

It is useful to keep in mind that Alzheimer's disease is a relative newcomer among the known degenerative brain diseases. In 1906, the German pathologist and neurologist Alois Alzheimer described a fifty-seven-year-old woman, Auguste D., who manifested progressive dementia (the inability to engage lucidly with other people and the loss of ability to conduct daily life), hallucinations (seeing or hearing things that are not there), and delusions (a false belief that things are occurring that are not). After Auguste D. passed away, Alzheimer succeeded in taking sections of her brain and putting stains on them so that he could identify the typical features of brain tissue, as well as the atypical. He observed what he called *amyloid plaques* (clumps of dark protein in the cortex and the hippocampus that may be seen by looking at the diseased brain through a microscope), and he described densely twisted bundles of *fibrils* (very fine fibers) that he called *neurofibrillary tangles*. I'll discuss these phenomena more later on.

Despite the fact that Alzheimer noted the signature signs of the disease in 1906, medical research in the disease lay dormant for nearly eighty years. Physicians treating the elderly accepted cognitive decline as a normal manifestation of the aging process partly because they lacked the appropriate research tools to properly understand it and to imagine a course of treatment. But in the late 1960s, Dr. Robert Katzman, a neurologist at Albert Einstein University and University of California–San Diego and one of my mentors, identified Alzheimer's as a potentially important and common disease. During the time that Dr. Katzman made this observation, many people did not recognize Alzheimer's disease and used terms like "hardening of the arteries" and "dementia." Almost all of those cases have turned out to be Alzheimer's disease.

This makes it likely that this disease is not new, only the recognition of it is relatively so.

But the changes that an Alzheimer's-affected brain undergoes were not understood until 1984, when Dr. George Glenner and Dr. C. W. Wong of the University of California–San Diego established that the appearance of amyloid plaque or the existence of a protein called *amyloid beta peptide* was the core constituent of a brain showing signs of Alzheimer's. These are described in detail in chapter 2. This finding was the foundation of many of the discoveries about Alzheimer's that have occurred in the last twenty years, providing further avenues of research among molecular biologists, geneticists, and brain pathologists. This was the real beginning of meaningful discussions about treatment of Alzheimer's disease and even, perhaps, its prevention.

Molecular biologists found that the amyloid protein came from a parent molecule called an *amyloid precursor protein* (APP). Their discovery of mutations of APP led to the initial understanding that such molecular changes trigger Alzheimer's disease. The first solid indication that these mutations were culprits came from research by a team headed by Henry Wisnewski in 1985. They found that people with Down syndrome, a genetic condition, have a high risk of acquiring early-onset Alzheimer's disease, beginning in their forties, and that Alzheimer's is a virtual certainty in Down syndrome individuals who live to their fifties. Using other breakthroughs in genetic engineering, scientists soon were able to develop mice with mutations that caused them to get Alzheimer's disease. Now, there is a whole subfield in Alzheimer's research devoted to understanding the mechanisms by which the brain produces amyloid, the cellular biology of amyloid processing, and the main reasons it causes toxic events, cell damage, and subsequent brain damage.

Now that you know the basics and the history of research relating to Alzheimer's, here are some of the things we doctors look for when we suspect Alzheimer's disease.

Alzheimer's patients go through three phases as they progress from mildly affected to advanced dementia. These phases are summarized in the following list.

Common Clinical Features of Alzheimer's Disease by Stage

Early stage. This is also called mild Alzheimer's. This stage of the disease is often mistaken for old age. The patient and the family will frequently dismiss the symptoms, attribute them to other reasons (for example, stress, preoccupation, old age, and so on), or not take the signs and symptoms seriously. Later, I will discuss more specifically the key things to look for if you think someone you know may be starting to manifest symptoms of Alzheimer's.

- **Memory**
  Poor recall of new information. People with Alzheimer's forget new facts and occurrences quickly, due to a loss of short-term memory. That is why they often repeat themselves. Long-term memory, or recall of things that happened in the distant past, is preserved.

- **Language**
  Dysnomia (impaired naming of objects). People with Alzheimer's have trouble recalling words and names, even ones very familiar to them, to a far greater degree than those who experience normal aging.

  Mild loss of fluency (language production). People with Alzheimer's tend to talk less over time.

- **Visuospatial**
  Misplacing objects. People with Alzheimer's lose glasses, keys, and other objects very frequently or put them in unusual, even inappropriate, places.

  Difficulty driving. People with Alzheimer's tend to have difficulty in perception and will make poor decisions while driving. This is a contentious issue that is often difficult for the family and the treating physician to deal with.

- **Behavioral**
  Depression. People with Alzheimer's are frequently depressed and withdrawn. Often early signs of Alzheimer's, such as loss of interest in activities or loss of initiative, are

mistaken for depression. However, when the depression is treated, cognitive impairment remains in people with this disease.

Anxiety. People with Alzheimer's often experience anxiety, sometimes related to short-term memory loss. They tend to feel uncertain in situations that are not routine or familiar.

Intermediate stage. This also referred to as moderate Alzheimer's. Symptoms become very apparent as Alzheimer's progresses. Often, this is the stage when family members seek care for their loved one with Alzheimer's, frequently because the symptoms have spread beyond simple memory loss and are starting to take a toll on all family members involved in the care of the person.

Memory

Remote memory. People with intermediate Alzheimer's begin to forget things in the distant past or to confuse the past with the present.

Language

Nonfluent (meaning loss of ability to produce language). Patients experience progressive and overt loss of language production.

Poor comprehension. Over time, Alzheimer's patients lose their ability to understand or follow conversations and instructions.

Visuospatial

Getting lost. Alzheimer's patients may begin to get lost in stores or places they have been many times before or even in their own neighborhood. They have a decreased sense of direction.

Behavioral

Delusions. People suffering Alzheimer's may begin to believe things that have not occurred have taken place, or vice versa. Examples of delusions include thinking something was stolen, when the Alzheimer's patient has simply lost the object. Another example is the delusion that people are conspiring to put the Alzheimer's person away or take his or her money. Yet another, more disturbing delusion is the idea that the spouse or caregiver is an impostor.

Depression. Alzheimer's patients often lose interest in participating in activities they once enjoyed. This can be either from the dementia or from depression. Sometimes it is difficult to tell. Alzheimer's patients tend to have less energy. This is frequently interpreted as depression.

Agitation. Verbal outbursts or physical threats for seemingly minor activities or requests such as bathing and eating. Often, patients become resistive to routine activities and may strike out at caregivers over seemingly minor things.

Sleep. Sleep disturbances are common complications of Alzheimer's disease progression and may include the loss of internal regulation of sleep, excessive medication use, sleep-disordered breathing, depression, and chronic bed rest. Related sleep disturbances like nocturnal wandering can increase caregiver burden.

Neurological

Frontal release signs. When Alzheimer's subjects are examined, they have features similar to infants such as a grasp reflex (a reflexive grabbing when something is placed in the palm) and a snout reflex (puckering of the lips in anticipation of being fed).

Extrapyramidal signs. Parkinson's disease–like features (stiffness, slowness of movement) may emerge at this stage, although they tend to be more pronounced in the advanced stage of the disease. When they are overt, we consider the possibility of other kinds of dementia.

Nonspecific gait disorder. People with Alzheimer's start to walk slower and may need assistance in walking.

Late stage. This is often referred to as severe Alzheimer's. By this stage, the disease has been present for many years, and most people with Alzheimer's disease are already in long-term care.

This is perhaps the most heartbreaking stage because at this point the people are dependent on others for care and survival. They lose their recognition of loved ones, even spouses of decades. They lose their ability to express their needs.

Memory

Short-term and long-term memories. Both are severely impacted. At this stage, people with Alzheimer's may no longer recognize loved ones or remember large segments of their lives.

Language

Lost language production. Patients with late-stage Alzheimer's often have lost language production to the point where their speech becomes largely unintelligible and their needs cannot be expressed clearly.

Behavioral

Agitation. Patients with Alzheimer's frequently become agitated. This might include physical aggression toward caregivers as well as resistance toward basic activities such as bathing and dressing.

Wandering. Patients with Alzheimer's frequently wander in the home or when unsupervised can wander in the neighborhood or even farther away.

Loss of insight. Late-stage Alzheimer's patients have no recognition or insight that there is anything wrong. When asked if they have Alzheimer's, they reply that they do not. This can be very distressing for families, especially when they try to point out a memory problem or an error in judgment; the person with Alzheimer's will flatly deny that anything is wrong. Because people with Alzheimer's lose insight, they can get agitated or paranoid as they are reacting to how people react to them, not understanding why other people react to them in certain ways.

Neurological

Incontinence. As Alzheimer's patients become very advanced, they lose control of bladder and bowel function.

This is one of the reasons people are placed into long-term care.

Frontal release signs. Infantile reflexes such as grasp, which are shed by the brain during normal childhood development, return with late-stage Alzheimer's.

Rigidity. Alzheimer's patients become increasingly slower and stiffer in movement.

Loss of gait. In the advanced stages, people with Alzheimer's are no longer able to walk and eventually cannot sit or hold themselves up.

Feeding and swallowing difficulties. In this stage, people forget to eat, forget to swallow, forget to chew, and pocket food (leave it in the mouth). The swallowing reflex becomes compromised, resulting in choking episodes and possibly pneumonia.

CASE STUDY

Anna Repeats Herself

Anna, an eighty-one-year-old woman, was brought to see me in my clinic at Sun Health Research Institute for an evaluation of memory loss of a progressive nature. The symptoms had been present for five years and were getting worse. Her memory loss originally took the form of a tendency to repeat questions and ideas. As the symptoms progressed, her daughter, Sylvia, reported that her mother was having trouble reasoning and was disoriented with regard to time, day, date, month, and year. Frequently, Anna did not understand where she was when outside the home. Sylvia described Anna as still experiencing anxiety and depression, which signified a personality change in her mother despite multiple courses of medication for depression. Anna now also tended to be verbally aggressive toward others, which was not her usual manner. In addition, Sylvia reported that her mother had begun to require supervision in dressing, bathing, and grooming—what we physicians call "functional decline"—and required reminders to change her clothes. Frequently, Anna would wear the same clothes repeatedly. In addition, she had become socially withdrawn.

During my evaluation, Anna told me that she cooked and cleaned her house, and how her husband didn't care, repeating the same statement eight times. She was also very upset when I examined her, because she did not comprehend why she was there. Throughout the visit, she had obvious difficulty finding words. Even without any other medical or neurological evaluations, all these indications made it obvious that she had classic Alzheimer's disease in the late mild/early moderate stage.

The simple fact is that not all forgetfulness is Alzheimer's. Additionally, with a lot of myths surrounding Alzheimer's disease, it is good to start with basic facts about what is true and not true about Alzheimer's disease specifically, and memory loss in general.

Alzheimer's Myths and Truths

Myth: All forgetfulness is Alzheimer's.

Not true: Some mild forgetfulness for names is expected as we age. Forgetfulness that portends Alzheimer's is characterized by rapid forgetting of present-day information or thoughts, such as forgetting appointments or repeating questions and statements.

Myth: All Alzheimer's includes forgetfulness.

True: One of the most salient features of Alzheimer's is short-term memory loss in the context of impairment in other aspects of living.

Myth: Alzheimer's is just old age.

Not true: Alzheimer's is a disease like heart disease, cancer, diabetes, and stroke, and can strike people as young as their forties or fifties while never affecting others of advanced age.

Myth: Dementia and Alzheimer's are the same thing.

Partially true: Alzheimer's is a type of dementia. So all Alzheimer's is dementia, but not every dementia is Alzheimer's.

Myth: I can't get Alzheimer's because it does not run in my family.

Not true: A family history of Alzheimer's certainly increases the risk but is not absolutely necessary to get Alzheimer's.

Myth: Memory loss can only occur from degenerative brain diseases.

Not true: There are medications that can cause or compound memory loss. Some metabolic conditions such as low blood sugar or low sodium can also exacerbate or mimic memory loss.

Myth: Alzheimer's disease can be diagnosed only at autopsy.

Partially true: This common myth is based on scientific opinions and criteria that are over twenty-two years old. Our science has progressed significantly since then; under the right circumstances, some doctors can diagnose Alzheimer's with greater than 90 percent accuracy during life. Thus, we are beginning to approach diagnosis not simply by excluding other conditions that can cause memory loss but by specifically identifying Alzheimer's with reasonably high accuracy. This is discussed further in chapter 19.

Not All Dementia Is Alzheimer's

Dementia is a category of disease. Saying a person has dementia is much like saying a person has cancer. Well, what kind of cancer? One could have leukemia, lymphoma, sarcoma, carcinoma, or melanoma, for example. Likewise, there are many types of dementia.

All dementias are characterized by cognitive decline (such as memory, orientation, and executive function [planning and executing tasks]) that affects daily life, but each type of dementia has different features that distinguish one kind from another. These differences are important, since they each require different diagnoses and treatment plans. These are summarized in the following list.

Types of Dementia

- **Alzheimer's disease.** Described earlier. It accounts for only half to two-thirds of all dementias. The remaining third includes the ones listed below.

- **Dementia with Lewy bodies (DLB).** This is the second most common type of dementia. It is characterized by progressive dementia coupled with slowness of movements and Parkinson's-like features (stiffness and problems walking), as well as clearly described hallucinations (particularly visual hallucinations: a tendency to see things that are not there and responding to stimuli from the person's own mind). People with DLB tend to have very rapidly progressing dementia and fluctuations of clarity followed by confusion. They tend to be very sensitive to medication that, although intended to improve symptoms, can make these sufferers worse. Interestingly, they may have a tendency to act out dreams that may precede the onset of the dementia. *Lewy bodies*, first identified by Frederic Lewy, are particular changes seen in brain cells and are most commonly associated with Parkinson's disease. What distinguishes DLB from Parkinson's is that Lewy bodies are concentrated in one part of the brain in Parkinson's, but widely distributed in DLB. Most sufferers of DLB have autopsy findings consistent with Alzheimer's disease.

- **Vascular dementia.** Strokes (cerebral thrombosis, hemorrhage, or cerebral embolism) can cause dementia, and such memory loss and cognitive decline can even start fairly abruptly following a stroke. *Vascular dementia* is characterized by changes identified on a brain scan such as a CT or an MRI. A clearly identified history of stroke is helpful although not always present. When examining a person with vascular dementia, an abnormal neurological examination is evident with focal weakness, loss of coordination, or trouble with balance. This type of dementia may not progress and can even improve with the right type of treatment.

- **Alzheimer's mixed with vascular dementia.** At autopsy, most individuals with vascular dementia have enough biological changes in their brains to fulfill the pathological criteria for Alzheimer's. Pure vascular dementia is far less common than is the mixture between Alzheimer's and stroke-induced vascular dementia. With mixed vascular/Alzheimer's, people can become worse even when they have not had another stroke. Some scientists and researchers believe that the causes of vascular dementia and Alzheimer's overlap. This will be discussed in chapter 7.

- **Frontotemporal dementia (FTD), or Pick's disease.** This is a relatively uncommon type of dementia, named for Arnold Pick, with an earlier age-of-onset (forty to sixty-five years old) than Alzheimer's disease. Many FTDs are linked to genetic mutations on chromosome 17 (scientists call these "the tauopathies"). More recently, scientists have discovered new mutations in a gene called progranulin. Symptoms include prominent language changes such as *anomia* (inability to name an object), *aphasia* (inability to generate or comprehend language), *echolalia* (a tendency to repeat everything said to them), and *perseverative speech* (a tendency to repeat a word or phrase in an obsessive manner, not realizing that they are doing so). Many patients suffering from this type of dementia lose social skills and display inappropriate behavior and judgment and lack of insight.

  One of my patients was a fifty-nine-year-old gentleman. His wife explained to me that he had started having trouble understanding what she was telling him about one to two years before their visiting my office. She also told me that he had tried to get out of the car when she was driving on the highway to their appointment with me. When I examined him, he was very restless and wandered about the room, standing and sitting repeatedly. Also during my examination of him, he could not converse well; he had trouble speaking as well as understanding. He had Pick's disease.

- **Parkinson's disease.** Parkinson's initially begins with movement problems and is clinically characterized by the presence of tremor (more commonly while the arms and legs are at rest and not in motion), *cogwheel rigidity* (stiff joints and limbs) and *bradykinesia* (slowness of movement). Parkinson's patients commonly have problems walking and have a tendency to fall. Dementia is common in advanced cases, although estimates of dementia prevalence vary widely— anywhere from 27 to 78 percent in some studies. Parkinson's dementia is different from Alzheimer's in that Parkinson's patients have slower recall, whereas Alzheimer's patients won't remember the same items at all. People with Parkinson's dementia tend to have more hallucinations. Both loss of mobility and loss of cognition contribute to the functional declines seen in Parkinson's dementia.

- **Huntington's disease.** This is a rare, inherited disease, detectable by genetic testing and brain scan, that has dramatic phenotypic characteristics, including *chorea* (uncontrollable writhing movements), depression, psychiatric changes, and dementia. Huntington's most commonly strikes individuals in their forties, fifties, and sixties, and has been genetically linked to mutations that occur on chromosome 4.

- **Other degenerative diseases.** Other diseases, such as progressive *supranuclear palsy*, a Parkinson's-like condition manifested by patients having significant balance problems and trouble moving their eyes; and *Lou Gehrig's disease* or *amyotrophic lateral sclerosis* (ALS), a degenerative disease that causes progressive atrophy (shrinkage) of muscles. Other degenerative brain diseases are associated with dementia. These are, for the most part, quite rare.

- **Dementias secondary to alcohol.** Alcohol-related dementia is well described and is linked to chronic consumption of alcohol for years. Keep in mind this is a distinct risk unrelated to mild alcohol use, which actually may protect against Alzheimer's disease. Alcohol-related dementias are subcategorized into different types. It is important to recognize, however, that acute confusion related to alcohol may also be due to a vitamin B₁ (thiamine) deficiency. Without proper treatment, thiamine deficiency from alcohol consumption can lead to a type of dementia called *Korsakoff dementia*, which is characterized by severe *anterograde amnesia* (inability to gather new memory), and *confabulation* (making things up to fill the gaps in memory). See chapter 12 for more on Korsakoff's and alcohol-related dementias.

- **Depression/pseudodementia.** Depression can masquerade as dementia, particularly in younger people. Depression-induced pseudodementia is distinguished from degenerative dementia by the sufferer's apathetic demeanor at diagnosis. Moreover, when such a patient gets treatment, his or her memory improves, unlike an Alzheimer's patient with depression, who may not necessarily experience an improvement in memory.

- **Normal pressure hydrocephalus (NPH).** This is an increasingly recognized condition that typically affects elderly individuals. It is characterized by walking and balance problems, followed by trouble controlling bladder function and memory loss. Important in the diagnosis of NPH is identification of abnormally large spaces in the brain called the *ventricles*; due to overaccumulation and reduced clearance of *cerebrospinal fluid* (CSF). NPH comes with good news: it is actually a treatable condition, and under the right circumstances, sufferers can expect a full recovery. A shunt that drains fluid from into the abdomen is implanted surgically and can be programmed to increase or decrease flow or pressure as needed. These programmable shunts have meant vast improvements in NPH therapy and hope for patients of this dementia.

- **Structural lesions.** Although rare, brain tumors can become symptomatic in the form of dementia. Twice, I have seen brain tumors present as dementia. Typically, they are large, near the middle of the brain, and involve the frontal lobe (front part of the brain). In both circumstances, the tumor was removed and the patient improved.

- **Endocrine disorders (hypothyroidism).** Thyroid deficiency is a well-known cause of dementia. It is less common than it used to be, since thyroid levels are routinely checked in medical practice. When a person has cognitive decline and dementia from thyroid deficiency, he or she tends to have other symptoms of hypothyroidism as well, including low energy level and weight gain.

- **Metabolic disorders.** Low sodium and low blood sugar at critically low levels can cause acute confusion and coma but are not common causes of dementia. We routinely check for low electrolytes in the course of a dementia evaluation.

- **Infections (for example, neurosyphillis, AIDS, CJD).** Before 1929, the most common form of dementia in the world was from syphilis. Since that time, with the advent of penicillin, dementia from syphilis has become quite rare in the Western world. It is still sometimes seen in urban clinics and can be a presenting sign of syphilis but mostly would follow the presence of other symptoms such as genital changes and a rash on the palms and the feet. Diagnosis of neurosyphillis involves a spinal tap to detect the infection in the central nervous system.

  Dementia from AIDS is a frequent disabling complication in advanced stages and is manifested by poor concentration and personality changes such as listlessness and indifference. *AIDS dementia complex*, as it is commonly called, affects the front part of the brain. It would not be a presenting feature of AIDS and occurs after AIDS symptoms have been present for long periods of time.

  Creutzfeldt-Jakob disease, or CJD, is the human equivalent of mad cow disease. In cows, it is called *bovine spongiform encephalopathy*; in sheep, it is called *scrapie*. In humans, it is acquired from transplantation or ingestion of infected human or cow tissue. Symptoms take years from time of infection to manifest. More specifically, the symptoms of the disease may start twenty years or more after exposure to the infected source. It was originally described in cannibals from New

Guinea who ate human remains, out of cultural beliefs. It is not limited to cannibals, but it does require exposure to the infection. The cause of CJD is neither a virus nor bacteria but rather a viruslike protein called a *prion*. CJD is characterized by rapid dementia and *myoclonus* (involuntary jerking of the body). Changes in spinal fluid and brain-wave studies (EEGs) can confirm a diagnosis; mention CJD or mad cow, however, and fear is struck in the heart of health-care workers, because there are no effective treatments. Once symptoms start, CJD is uniformly fatal and life expectancy is less than one year. Thankfully, this is still quite rare, and infection from eating infected meat is not only exceedingly infrequent but still quite controversial as regards its being a definitive cause of this disease.

- **Medication effects.** Many medications, prescribed and over-the-counter alike, may adversely affect memory. These include preparations for sleep, such as anything that has "PM" in the name; some antihistamines for allergies, such as diphenhydramine (Benadryl and other brands); certain bladder medications, such as oxybutinin (Ditropan); and some epilepsy medications, such as phenobarbital. In fact, many drugs affect cognitive function when taken in excess, including such sedatives as diazepam (Valium). Ask your doctor if the medications you are taking could affect your memory.

How Do You Know You Are Getting Alzheimer's?

Toward the end of this book, in chapter 19, are a few questionnaires that you can take if you are concerned that you or a loved one is developing Alzheimer's. Early Alzheimer's is often mistaken for old age. Loved ones and friends often overlook the misplacing of keys as simple inattention. But if such events of memory loss become repetitive or obvious, consider seeking medical attention. It is important to think of Alzheimer's and dementia as you would any disease: you *need* to seek medical attention.

Beyond this awareness, the following telltale signs indicate that something is really wrong. These ten warning signs are also seen at the Alzheimer's Association Web site (www. alz.org).

Ten Warning Signs of Alzheimer's

- **Memory loss that affects job skills.** If you are laid off, keep moving from job to job, or are demoted because you cannot remember tasks or have trouble learning new tasks, you may be exhibiting signs of early Alzheimer's.

  Once I had a patient who was a battleship repairman. He was a master craftsman who had to follow and understand very complex diagrams in order to repair battleships. His first sign of Alzheimer's was difficulty in reading diagrams and following instructions on complicated repair jobs. These problems and difficulties ultimately led to his losing his job.

  Another patient of mine was an executive who noticed that she was having trouble understanding, tracking, and remembering her account spreadsheets and business plans. This change in her work habits alarmed her and forced her into retirement earlier than planned. These symptoms were her first sign of Alzheimer's.

  Yet another of my patients was a nurse anesthetist and a faculty member of a nearby nursing school. She had an important job, being responsible for the nurse anesthesia program at that school. She ended up on disability because she lost her ability to develop curricula, teach, plan, and administrate the very programs she had created. First, she was put on part-time work status and ultimately on disability. Her Alzheimer's was positively diagnosed at the age of fifty-nine.

- **Difficulty performing familiar tasks.** These can include cooking, check writing and other bookkeeping, supermarket shopping, and home maintenance. Simply put, if the person is struggling to do a familiar task or has given it up altogether, suspect Alzheimer's.

  One of my patients had been a general contractor. He could build or repair anything in the home. His first sign that he had Alzheimer's was that he was starting a lot of home-repair projects but either not finishing them or taking weeks to finish what in the past would have taken him mere hours or days to complete.

Another patient of mine used to be a great cook. She was admired and beloved by friends and family alike because of her culinary skills. Her first sign of Alzheimer's was her inability to follow recipes. Her husband reported that the taste of her cooking was not like it used to be.

Yet another of my patients used to be able to calculate his taxes by hand every year (I certainly can't do that). His Alzheimer's was signaled by his trouble following the line-by-line instructions and his loss of the ability to calculate his taxes with pencil and paper.

Another of my patients was formerly a music conductor and an avid musician. He could hear every instrument in his head when he conducted and would memorize entire musical scores. The onset of Alzheimer's caused him to lose the ability to read and follow the music sheets when he was conducting. Furthermore, he could no longer memorize an entire score.

The recurrent theme here is that all of these people were reported to have difficulty doing tasks they had done not only repeatedly but well in the past.

- **Problems with language, especially words and names.** This is a common complaint in Sun City and among seniors in general, so let me make a distinction here. If you have not seen someone you know for twenty years and you can't remember his/her name, that is merely a "senior moment." That kind of trouble remembering names probably does not represent the beginning Alzheimer's disease. However, when it is Alzheimer's disease, the word-finding difficulty can be much worse. Recently I saw a patient with Alzheimer's who called her spouse by her son's name.

- **Substituting one word for another.** This phenomenon is called *paraphasia*. In paraphasia, the concept is understood but one word is substituted for another. For example, a person with Alzheimer's might refer to a wooden pencil as a pen. In descriptive paraphasia, the person describes the object in place of naming it. For instance, someone with descriptive paraphasia might call a watchband "the part that keeps it on the wrist." Both paraphasia and descriptive paraphasia are common in Alzheimer's. Often a caregiver is forced to play the guessing game to determine what the person with Alzheimer's is talking about or whom the individual is referring For example, the woman I mentioned above called a "watch" a "clock" and called the tip of the pen "the ink." She made other mistakes of naming as well.

- **Disorientation to time and place.** This includes trouble tracking days and dates. In Sun City, many of my patients hide their deficit by saying, "Doc, I am retired—I don't have to know that." If the person is getting ready for church, however, thinking it is Sunday but it is Wednesday, then it is time to worry. Many of my patients suffering from Alzheimer's look at the newspaper or calendar daily to know what is the day, date, month, or year. Regularly I ask the year or other items of orientation. One gentleman replied 1947 for the year, when it was 2007.

- **Poor or decreased judgment.** Examples of decreased judgment might include a person's diminished ability to track investments, or trusting others to do it for him or her without knowing them well. This might manifest itself in an increased vulnerability to telemarketers, door-to-door solicitation, or giving away money without having a full accounting of the recipient's finances. When the dementia gets worse, often there is paranoia. People with Alzheimer's might believe that family members are conspiring to take their money away even when things are explained to them. They may become mistrustful of those who had been trustworthy.

- **Problems with abstract thinking.** People with Alzheimer's have trouble grasping abstract thoughts. This can include learning new tasks or trouble comprehending nuanced topics such as poetry, metaphors, or difficult story lines in books and movies.

- **Misplacing things.** This is a manifestation of short-term memory loss. In normal aging, misplacing things is an infrequent event. With Alzheimer's disease, it can become so frequent to the point that families make looking for objects such as keys and glasses a part of their daily routine. One man I know spends all his daytime hours trying to find objects that his wife, my patient with Alzheimer's, misplaces.

- **Changes in mood or behavior.** Many people with Alzheimer's manifest depression and/or anxiety. This is often identified by loss of interest or by complaints of fatigue. Sometimes, normally social individuals will become socially withdrawn at the onset of clinical Alzheimer's.

- **Changes in personality.** Frequently, families comment about a senior's increased irritability and hostility toward loved ones. Mainly, they have a "shorter fuse." Alternatively, people with Alzheimer's may become passive, docile, or complacent.

  Following is an example of personality change manifested as irritability and hostility:

  Patient: "Dear, when is my appointment?"
  Spouse: "I have told you five times already. It is tomorrow morning!"
  Patient: "No, you haven't! You are lying. I would remember if you told me. . . ."

- **Loss of initiative.** Patients with Alzheimer's disease often lose interest in activities they formerly enjoyed, such as hobbies, reading, or chores, and prefer to become sedentary. Loss of initiative is often mistaken for depression.

If you recognize these signs in yourself or someone you know or love, then maybe it is time to see your doctor about it. Ultimately, it is important to recognize the symptoms and not ascribe them to old age or stress. What to do about Alzheimer's is discussed in more detail in chapter 19.

From Normal Aging to Alzheimer's:
Mild Cognitive Impairment

People do not go from normal one day to Alzheimer's the next. The transition to Alzheimer's disease passes through an intermediate state called *mild cognitive impairment* (MCI). Metaphorically, MCI is the chest pain before the heart attack, the colon polyp before the colon cancer, the mole before the melanoma, the slightly elevated blood sugar before the diabetes. It is the intermediate state between being normal and having Alzheimer's.

MCI is characterized by subtle but measurable memory problems, and those who suffer from MCI have memory problems that are greater than typical for their age. Currently, this is a topic of intense debate in the medical community because many top researchers and clinicians believe that if intervention occurs at this intermediate stage, Alzheimer's disease might be delayed or arrested completely. Here are the clinical criteria for MCI:

- Memory difficulties are attested to by a patient and/or the patient's family. These lapses can interfere with the patient's ability to adapt and function in daily life.

- Selective memory lapses are measured by neuropsychological tests (extensive paper-and-pencil tests administered by trained professionals called *neuropsychologists*) while other brain functions register normal or near-normal.

- Although the patient's ability to complete complex tasks may be compromised, other activities of daily living, such as traveling, paying bills, and balancing a checkbook, remain unaffected.

- The patient is not demented. The distinguishing feature that separates MCI from Alzheimer's or dementia is the absence of functional impairment. Generally, such people are still getting along through life.

MCI is a common condition that may or may not be an omen of the decline in memory that accompanies the onset of Alzheimer's. Until very recently, doctors and scientists have not had a consistent definition for this stage of impairment, making it difficult to estimate how common MCI really is. In long-term community-based studies of elderly subjects, we estimate that between 2 and 5 percent of people will convert from a cognitively normal state to dementia each year. Similarly, the incidence of cognitive impairment without dementia in these studies rises rapidly with age, reaching 2.4 to 7.9 percent by ages eighty to eighty-four. When we apply a strict definition to MCI with rigorous clinical and scientific criteria to back it up, then studies have reported the incidence of MCI to average around 1 percent per year. The time taken to "convert" from normal cognition to MCI and from MCI to dementia is the measurement that has been used to gauge the rate of cognitive change.

Although it's a crude measure of the progress of disease, this rate of conversion is also important because it helps us measure the efficacy of various drugs. In addition, it helps us predict the rate of the progress of the disease in a population that is converting to Alzheimer's in precipitous numbers. Further, as a transitional state between normal aging and Alzheimer's disease, it is a barometer of risk for developing Alzheimer's. Between 10 and 15 percent of all individuals diagnosed with MCI convert to Alzheimer's every year. In fact, there is a 50 percent conversion after five years and more than a 90 percent conversion after ten years.

In population-based epidemiological studies—that is, studies that are done on the general population rather than in a defined community—one-quarter of all MCI cases revert to a normal cognitive state, about half remain unchanged, and another quarter become demented within two years. In contrast, clinical studies of subjects with identified MCI with prominent memory loss are much more likely to convert to dementia, and reversals are rare. In fact, someone with MCI who has mainly memory loss is twenty-six times more likely to develope Alzheimer's than is an age-matched normal individual.

Although it is a very strong indicator, not all MCI is a prelude to Alzheimer's. Infrequently, MCI can be a marker of stress, depression, hearing loss, heart disease, nutritional deficiency, sleep disturbance, or inactivity. I have seen sleep apnea that was so severe that it caused memory impairment. Once it was treated, memory loss drastically improved.

CASE STUDY

Old Age or MCI?

Heidi, an eighty-year-old woman with sixteen years of education, was referred to me for evaluation of memory loss. The patient articulately described her situation in her own words. She noted memory loss, such as a tendency to leave items cooking on the stove—she had burned many pans as a result. She said she had trouble remembering tasks, and forgot why she was doing things. She denied a tendency to repeat herself. She noted that she had become more withdrawn and been slightly depressed, indicating personality and mood changes. There was also a functional decline, as manifested by her admission to a tendency to procrastinate, which she never used to do. She got lost while driving and had a decreased sense of direction. When I examined her and tested her orientation, there was some disorientation to place. She also noted that she was having trouble finding words and names in conversations. She had not decreased her pursuit of pleasurable activities, however, and denied the presence of hallucinations or delusions. Her memory screening showed that she had difficulty recalling a name and address that I asked her to remember after a five-minute delay. The rest of her neurological exam was normal.

Further evaluation with extensive neuropsychological tests (the paper-and-pencil test described on page 32 and further in chapter 19) revealed a significant problem with memory but no problems in other areas tested. She therefore had MCI.

If MCI can present its symptoms so subtly, how can you tell if you have it or not? Diagnosing MCI is often challenging and is best done with neuropsychological tests. These tests are paper-and-pencil memory tests that often take several hours to complete. Essentially, they are mental gymnastics.

One study from the University of California–Irvine found that using simple tests of memory (remembering a list of items) was 98 percent accurate in distinguishing MCI from early Alzheimer's, and 97 percent accurate in distinguishing normal memory for age from MCI. These rates show that getting tested is accurate and worthwhile. Anyone experiencing symptoms of MCI, whether it's you or someone you know, should seek an evaluation that includes blood tests and imaging.

Treating MCI is controversial, and experts have not reached a consensus that treatment with the medications available today is productive. Some physicians believe that the drugs used to treat Alzheimer's could be used to treat MCI. However, recent studies only show modest benefit with most Alzheimer's drugs currently on the market. Only donepezil (Aricept) has been shown to delay conversion to Alzheimer's and, even then, this is a delay of only six to twelve months, not a long-term preventative measure. With so little agreement in the medical community, the decision to treat MCI is one that should take place between the patient and a physician who has the most up-to-date knowledge about this condition.

Real MCI is the window a person has to address long-term life plans, like legal and financial matters, and family discussions about caretaking. Avoiding addressing the symptoms of MCI may result only in confronting a crisis situation later once the ravages of Alzheimer's have fully manifested themselves.

When Is It Old Age and When Is It Dementia?

Not all memory loss is Alzheimer's. Conversely, Alzheimer's is not simply old age. It is important to realize that most memory lapses in people over age fifty are likely benign. The term coined for benign forgetfulness is *age-associated memory impairment.*

Forgetting where you parked the car at the mall or your grand-child's name may just be old age, but forgetting that you have been to the mall or forgetting that your grandchild is related to you is more serious. There is a difference. In the early stages, such lapses may be subtle, and the person can cover for these changes. How-ever, every case of dementia reaches a point where it can no longer be confused with old age. The table below summarizes the differ-ence between the two.

When Is Memory Loss Normal Aging and When Is It Alzheimer's?

ABILITY	NORMAL AGING	ALZHEIMER'S DEMENTIA
Independent activities of daily living (for example, driving, finances, telephone, shopping)	Preserved	Impaired early and worsens with disease progression
Personal-care activities of daily living (for example, dressing, grooming, bathing)	Preserved	Impaired as disease progresses
Language	Occasional word-finding difficulties	Frequent loss or misapplication of words
Complaints of memory loss	Frequent, particularly for words and names	Does not complain of memory loss
Awareness of memory loss	Preserved	Impaired
Social skills	Intact	Preserved early, lost later
Memory for recent events	Details preserved	Either recall is lost altogether or details are lost

(continued)

When Is Memory Loss Normal Aging and
When Is It Alzheimer's? *(continued)*

ABILITY	NORMAL AGING	ALZHEIMER'S DEMENTIA
Performance on cognitive testing	Preserved in all areas	Impaired in memory and other areas such as orientation, language, executive function
Orientation	Preserved, does not get lost, tracks days, dates, and time	Impaired; gets lost even in own neighborhood, has trouble with dates and time
Able to learn new skills	Slow but preserved	Lost. Cannot learn new technologies such as programming a remote control or operating a new appliance

Final Thoughts and Recommendations

- Know and pay attention to the telltale signs of memory loss.
- Alzheimer's is a disease; it is not simply old age.
- Alzheimer's is a type of dementia.
- Not all dementia is Alzheimer's.
- Don't ignore signs of cognitive decline; if they are apparent in you or someone you love, seek medical attention.

2

Alzheimer's and the Brain

A brain from a person with Alzheimer's does not look the same as that of a person who died of "old age." It is much more shrunken. It can be up to one-third smaller and lighter because of the shrinkage (called *atrophy*). When the brain shrinks so dramatically, the spaces on the outside of the brain (called *sulci*) get farther apart.

A lot of changes occur in the Alzheimer's patient's brain. Some changes happen one at a time and some occur all at once and are not a normal part of the process of aging.

Among the changes in the brain of someone with Alzheimer's seen at autopsy are the following:

- Excessive shrinkage of the brain (atrophy, as described previously).

- Loss of the brain cells. The main type of brain cells that are lost are called *neurons*. The neurons responsible for memory are particularly vulnerable.

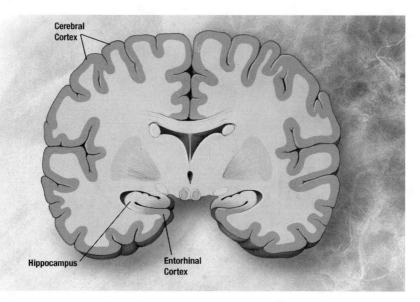

Cerebral
Cortex

Hippocampus

Entorhinal
Cortex

Preclinical slice of a brain of a person without Alzheimer's disease. There is no
atrophy (or shrinkage) and the folds of the brain, called gyri, are close together.

- Loss of the connections between nerve cells (called *synapses*),
  meaning that brain cells relay less information among one
  another
- Accumulation of senile plaques (described in detail further
  on).
- Accumulation of neurofibrillary tangles (described in detail
  further on).
- Accumulation of inflammation in the brain.

The first three changes in the brain can be caused by any number of pathologies. In the case of Alzheimer's, however, they are
the result of subtle changes in the structure of brain cells. These
changes are the direct result of the presence and accumulation of
amyloid, leading to what are called *neuritic senile plaques*. The
appearance of these plaques and the neurofibrillary tangles that
follow or accompany them are the signature traits of Alzheimer's
disease.

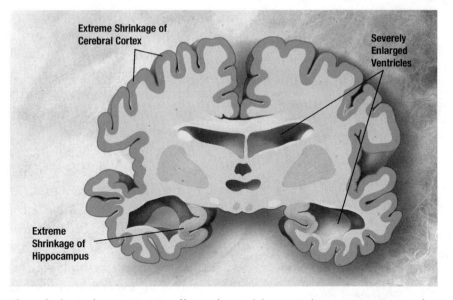

Slice of a brain from a person suffering from Alzheimer's disease. Apparent is a lot of atrophy, and the gyri are wide apparent.

There is no single culprit in Alzheimer's. Rather, Alzheimer's is the result of a specific cascade of events that lead to the destruction or profound impairment of brain cells and their functioning. To understand this cascade, you must first have some grasp of the molecules involved and the cell structures affected.

What Is a Plaque and Why Is It Important?

The figure on page 38 shows a slice of brain belonging to someone who died with Alzheimer's. In the middle is a dark cloud: that is a plaque. It is not the same plaque that your dentist scrapes off your teeth, nor is it the kind that builds up in arteries and heart to cause a heart attack or stroke.

This is brain plaque, and it is made up of cellular waste that has accumulated immediately outside the ends of cells. This waste is

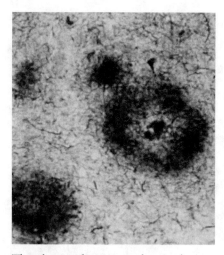

The plaques that accumulate in the brain of people suffering from Alzheimer's disease. This is an accumulation of an abnormal type of protein called amyloid.

made up of proteins called amyloid and inflammatory molecules called *cytokines,* as well as of other components of cellular breakdown. In other words, plaque is made of all the debris from dying or dead cells.

At the heart of the plaque is a protein called *amyloid,* which is a by-product of protein processing. Amyloid is a slice of a larger molecule called *amyloid precursor protein* (APP). When APP degrades normally during our bodies' everyday upkeep of cells, an enzyme called *alpha-secretase* splits the APP molecule in the middle of the amyloid molecule, like scissors cutting cleanly through thread. This enables the protein to be easily processed as a waste product as part of normal maintenance inside and outside of brain cells.

In Alzheimer's, for reasons we don't entirely understand, alpha-secretase becomes less active. This allows other enzymes (called *beta-* and *gamma-secretase*) to hijack the normal course of events. These enzymes produce the amyloid fragments that accumulate in the brain of Alzheimer's patients. These fragments are not as amenable to easy disposal as waste is.

Normal amyloid is a protein molecule comprised of forty amino acids (building blocks of proteins) aligned in a specific sequence. This molecule is generally cleared from the brain in much the same way that all cell waste is cleared away. Abnormal amyloid, called *beta-amyloid protein,* is forty-two amino acids long and is not cleared away. When it builds up in the brain, it causes a lot of collateral damage. Basically, beta-amyloid protein is unable to be cut out of APP like pieces of thread, because it is very sticky and clumps together easily. It clumps together like lint, and once it does so, it is not easily removed or dissolved.

Amyloid plaques are created when beta-amyloid protein sets off a chain of chemical events that leads to the build up of these pieces of amyloid, which then clump together into an amyloid plaque. As the plaques accumulate in the brain, they interfere with the normal processing of brain cells. This is depicted in the figures below.

Cell Membrane / APP Molecule

Cell Interior

The APP molecule is partly inside the brain cell but most of it is outside. It is a long, threadlike protein.

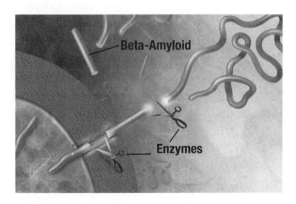

Beta-Amyloid

Enzymes

In Alzheimer's disease, the APP molecule is spliced with scissorlike proteins called beta- and gamma-secretase. The threadlike protein that is cut out between the scissors is beta-amyloid protein.

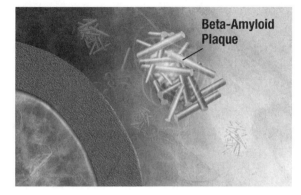

Beta-Amyloid Plaque

This beta-amyloid protein clumps together readily and forms the foundation of the plaque. These plaques accumulate outside brain cells but are toxic to the brain environment.

How Plaques Damage Brain Cells

As you can see, beta-amyloid protein is created from the larger protein APP. Once this occurs, beta-amyloid protein aggregates together to form fibrils (strands) and then sheets, a process called *fibrillization*. These events are important first steps that lead to the formation of plaques (as depicted in the illustration on page 39).

Once the plaque matures, its presence leads to many events that damage brain cells. Cells in the brain perceive the amyloid plaques as foreign, and so an immune response occurs, just as what happens when you have an infection. Plaques cause brain cells that surround the dying neurons (called *glia*) to secrete other chemicals that cause some brain cells to become too excited (literally, *excitotoxicity*). Plaques can also cause *free radicals* to be released. Free radicals are small molecules that are by-products of chemical reactions that can damage the structures of the cells.

Since the aggregation of beta-amyloid protein into fibrils and the subsequent formation of amyloid plaques are widely thought to be important steps in the pathogenesis of Alzheimer's, these processes are potential targets for therapy and drugs that may intervene and stop development of amyloid plaques.

Tangles

Another change that occurs in the brain of Alzheimer's patients is the accumulation of proteins called *neurofibrillary tangles*. These occur within the brain's neurons, rather than outside them where plaque develops. Neurons have arms called *axons*. Inside these axons are parallel proteins called *microtubules*. Just as railroad tracks that are kept together with railroad ties, microtubules are kept together with proteins called *tau*.

In Alzheimer's, these tau proteins undergo a biochemical change called *hyperphosphorylation*. This leads to the tau getting all jumbled up, which leads to the microtubules also becoming ensnarled, in a process called *paired helical filaments* (PHF).

Researchers have learned that even before tau start clumping together with microtubules to form tangles, the structures inside the brain cells have already begun to change: when microtubule proteins become misshapen, they start to clump, causing all the molecules that move along the microtubules to back up because they cannot get past the clog.

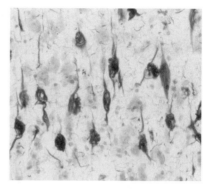

The teardrop shapes are dead brain cells called neurons that refilled with neurofibrillary tangles.

Ultimately, this leads to the neuron's being choked off, which causes an interruption in the communication chain that the affected neuron is part of. The photograph on the right shows the remnants of a brain cell taken from a brain autopsy. The wispy fibers are the neurofibrillary tangles.

In the course of Alzheimer's disease, attacks on both the inside and the outside of each brain cell are thus left unchecked, as is depicted in the figure below.

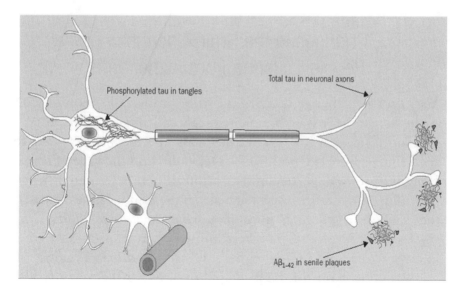

This is a depiction of a brain cell called a neuron. Inside the neuron (the left side of the picture) are threadlike protein inclusions called phosphorylated tau. This tau accumulates and becomes neurofibrillary tangles that disrupt internal cellular function and eventually contribute to cellular demise.

Loss of Synapse Leads to Loss of Communication among Cells

Synaptic damage is a telltale sign in Alzheimer's pathology as well. Synapses are the hands and feet of brain cells that connect to other brain cells so that they can communicate with one another. In Alzheimer's, the level of damage synapses have sustained is in direct proportion to the level of observed dementia. In other words, the greater the loss of synapses, the worse the dementia. Recently, researchers have suggested that the damage they were seeing might be caused by free-floating clumps of amyloid rather than by amyloid plaques. If amyloid in this smaller form is at play in synapse damage, it shifts the research focus to an earlier point in the Alzheimer's cascade. Then the object of treatment becomes trying to arrest amyloid accumulation itself, long before plaques begin to form. This possibility falls in line with the whole mission of Alzheimer's research. That is, we need to look earlier and earlier at the chain of events that lead to memory loss, to develop effective therapy strategies and targets.

Changes in the Brain Chemistry of People Suffering from Alzheimer's

Yet another change occurs in the brains of people with Alzheimer's: the loss of brain chemicals called *neurotransmitters*. Neurotransmitters are brain chemicals specifically designed to send signals between brain cells. Depending on the type of signal being transmitted, particular neurotransmitters act differently and are assigned to perform specific tasks in the brain. These transmitters include *dopamine, norepinephrine, histamine, glutamate, glycine,* and *serotonin*. The best known neurotransmitter that is known to be lost in Alzheimer's is *acetylcholine*. The loss of acetylcholine is one of the principal reasons for the memory loss that characterizes Alzheimer's disease.

Acetylcholine is the chemical substrate for memory. That means it is the chemical the brain uses to facilitate storage of memory.

The current thinking is that memory is encoded onto proteins. Acetylcholine is the chemical that facilitates this process to occur. Without acetylcholine, memory is not laid down in the brain. In other words, the new memories are never saved to begin with, and recollection becomes lost. In Alzheimer's disease, acetylcholine is lost because the brain cells that produce it die in the early stages of the disease. One of the earliest and most significant discoveries in the pathogenesis (understanding of the causes of the brain changes that occur) of Alzheimer's disease was the identification of this decline in levels of acetylcholine. In the more than thirty years since this discovery, the scientific evidence supporting it has grown. This research paved the way for the development of the very first Alzheimer's medications.

Many of the current medications used to treat Alzheimer's work by preventing the breakdown of acetylcholine in the brain. The longer that acetylcholine is produced and stays in the brain, the more it is available for use in the production of memory, which leads to more memories being preserved.

Adding It All Up

In summary, the brain undergoes a cascade of events in Alzheimer's that leads to mental decline and the inability to function in everyday life. Understanding this chain of events can help us to develop interventions that may ameliorate the symptoms or stop the progress of this disease. The next questions to ponder are: Can any of these physiological changes be prevented? Can the cascade be stopped before it has even begun? The answer is outlined in upcoming chapters.

Final Thoughts and Recommendations

Some of the pathological changes in the brain of someone with Alzheimer's include:

- Excessive atrophy (shrinkage) of the brain

- Loss of cholinergic neurons (the brain cells responsible for memory)
- Loss of synapses, the connections between nerve cells
- Presence and accumulation of neurofibrillary tangles inside the neurons that eventually lead to loss of normal functioning within brain cells
- Amyloid accumulation and deposition on the outside of the neurons, which clump together in a fashion that leads to the formation of the senile plaque

3

Is Preventing Alzheimer's Disease Really Possible?

Alzheimer's is not a minor problem that affects a few elderly. It is a major health crisis, one that affects a large segment of our society, costing billions of dollars a year to treat and in lost income. Following are the statistics for the occurrence of Alzheimer's in this country as we know them. They are sobering.

Alzheimer's in America: A Snapshot

- Approximately 5 million Americans currently suffer from Alzheimer's.

- Seven of every 100 people over the age of sixty-five will develop Alzheimer's. By 2010, that number will be one in ten Americans over age sixty-five.

- Every year, 100,000 people die from Alzheimer's disease.

- It is estimated that between 14 and 16 million Americans will have Alzheimer's by the year 2050.

- There are 1.5 million residents in nursing facilities nation-wide. Over half of them have dementia.

- Alzheimer's disease alone accounts for 40 percent of all long-term-care insurance claims. In less than five years, it is expected to account for 60 percent.

- Sadly, more than two-thirds of patients suffering from Alzheimer's are diagnosed when the disease has progressed beyond the mildest stages.

- Ten percent of the people over the age of sixty-five have Alzheimer's. This increases to between 32 and 47 percent by age eighty-five.

- The number of people with Alzheimer's doubles every five years after the age of sixty-five.

- The cost of caring for someone with Alzheimer's is almost double that of caring for someone who doesn't have the disease.

The Population Is Aging

By the middle of this century, there will be over *two billion* people over the age of sixty worldwide. The population boom in the aged is skyrocketing.

The statistics listed previously are impressive, but they are nothing less than staggering when we step back and look at the last century. In 1900, the average life expectancy in the United States was forty-seven years. In 2000, it was seventy-seven years. And today's best estimates put the average life expectancy in the United States above ninety by the year 2100!

Not only is the over-sixty crowd booming, but the number of very aged is rising, too. In fact, nonagenerians (those who are ninety plus) and centenarians (those who are one hundred plus) are the fastest growing segment of the U.S. population. This has far-reaching implications: it means that more seniors will be vulnerable to developing Alzheimer's than ever before.

Part of this aging trend is due to the decline in the infant mortality rate, which plummeted in the wake of important public health improvements such as sanitation infrastructure and universal vaccination practices. No longer do frequent outbreaks of measles, mumps, rubella, tuberculosis, plaque, and smallpox ravage large segments of the population. These days, people are less likely to die in younger life from a variety of conditions than were their forebears. Paradoxically, since age is the biggest risk factor for Alzheimer's, the very medical breakthroughs that resulted in these longer life expectancies have created a demographic time bomb for Alzheimer's disease.

The current cost of care for those affected by Alzheimer's disease is exploding. As the following list indicates, costs presently exceed $100 billion annually in the United States and are expected to increase proportionately with the incidence of Alzheimer's. Sweden's Karolinska Institute put the global cost at $156 billion in 2003, meaning now and in the foreseeable future, the United States shoulders the lion's share of Alzheimer's disease and the cost of caring for its sufferers. In fact, here in the United States, in terms of cost, Alzheimer's ranks third nationwide, behind only heart disease and cancer.

These estimates are so high because the costs of care go far above and beyond medication costs, much of it tied to institutional-based care, such as long-term care facilities. The current cost estimates of Alzheimer's care include:

- $60 billion a year shouldered by American businesses.

- $24.6 billion in health care for people with Alzheimer's.

- $36.5 billion in business costs for employees who are caregivers to people with Alzheimer's disease.

- $64 million for Employee Assistance Program usage.

- $18,408 per patient per year for mild Alzheimer's, $30,096 per patient per year for moderate Alzheimer's, and $36,132 per patient per year for severe Alzheimer's.

- Long-term care costs of $40,000 to $60,000 per year. In a survey conducted in 2003 by the General Electric Financial Company, the average annual cost of nursing home care was $57,700.

- Families paying cash to cover what Medicare, Medicaid, or long-term care insurance does not cover.

- The direct cost of caring for an Alzheimer's patient from diagnosis to death of $174,000, as reported by the American Health Assistance Foundation. Some estimate that Alzheimer's patients/families spend more than $200,000 for care over the remainder of the patient's life.

- Fifty percent more spent by people with Alzheimer's in a managed care plan over those in the plan who don't have Alzheimer's, as shown in a study of a managed Medicare plan. Approximately 477 hours of care/supervision per month are required by patients with Alzheimer's.

Prevention versus Cure: The Preferred Intervention

The past decade has given us a sobering lesson in the difficulty of reversing or slowing the cognitive and functional decline accompanying Alzheimer's. Depending on the degree of impairment, preserving the intellectual skills of someone after the onset of Alzheimer's disease may be a laudable goal, but not a realistic one. The simple truth is that our present treatments for Alzheimer's improve symptoms for a while (see chapter 19 for more details), but they can't significantly slow the disease. And even if the therapies improve, they will only compound the problem: if we succeed in slowing the progress of the disease, we will increase life expectancy among people with Alzheimer's, thereby also increasing the prevalence of Alzheimer's in the elderly population. From a public health perspective, our goal needs to be to *prevent or delay* the onset of the disease entirely. Prevention or delay would actually decrease the prevalence of Alzheimer's, a far more feasible and desirable goal.

There is another concern. After the decades-long presymptomatic and latent stages of the disease, comes the far shorter mild cognitive impairment (MCI) stage. Unfortunately, treatments for MCI have not yet translated into a significant delay in the onset of full-blown Alzheimer's disease. If the therapies in this book work, intervening in an individual's thirties through sixties could slow the progression and accumulation in the latent phase, thus delaying the appearance of symptoms in later years. Such preventive action could either keep a person from getting Alzheimer's altogether or shorten the course of the disease, lengthening the symptom-free life stage.

The Prevention of Alzheimer's Is a Top Public Health Priority

The statistics presented in this chapter amount to an urgent call for health and aging research that focuses on prevention rather than postsymptomatic intervention. We need to find ways to help the growing elderly population maintain its cognitive health into old age by delaying the onset of impairment and by reducing the total number of people affected by dementia.

As researchers, we need to continue rigorously investigating strategies for the prevention of Alzheimer's disease and dementia. Our goal is to lengthen the time before the onset of either Alzheimer's or MCI. If we can get Alzheimer's and MCI to begin at only eighty or ninety years of age, instead of at sixty or seventy, this will constitute a real breakthrough.

There is also a financial impetus for seeking ways to delay or prevent the onset of Alzheimer's. Research has shown that achieving even a modest delay—one year, in this case—would reduce the prevalence of Alzheimer's by 5 percent by the year 2030. That's 200,000 people who wouldn't get Alzheimer's at all. And if interventions could delay the onset of the disease by two years, after fifty years there would be 2 million fewer cases annually than are projected now. In economic terms, achieving that same two-year delay would result in a *$20 billion savings annually.* Frankly, we can't afford *not* to pursue prevention.

From both a personal and a public health perspective, focusing on prevention is the obvious choice. But the ultimate public health conundrum—you can't measure how many people didn't get sick who otherwise might have—makes prevention a tricky goal compared with cures, which are easier to count. Counting healthy individuals is in fact achievable, however: when the long-term care industry is struggling to fill beds it once filled with Alzheimer's patients, we will know that we have succeeded. We are a long way from that day. But we hope that the advances outlined in this book will move us all one step closer to it.

More than a decade ago, a researcher used statistical analysis in coronary heart disease to show that primary intervention using medication and lifestyle interventions (in this case, before heart attacks had occurred) would yield the highest proportions of disease-free individuals. In other words, the researcher found that preventing heart disease in the first place, which would reduce the likelihood of heart attacks, would actually be more economical than treating the cardiac damage that occurs during and after a heart attack. The analysis by that researcher also suggested that intensive medical treatment after disease onset—even at the earliest possible point—can reduce death (called *mortality* in medical terms) and complications or disability from disease (called *morbidity* in medical terms), but eventually increases the prevalence of the disease, thereby adding to the total burden of disease in the larger population.

If we don't pursue prevention as a target, we will witness health-care costs spinning even further out of control as our society shells out more and more money for terminal care and institution-based care (such as long-term care, assisted living, group homes, and dementia units), leaving less and less for research and development of new drugs or pursuing new avenues of research. Not only is such an approach reckless from a humanitarian perspective, it is economically unsustainable as well. Facing the tripling of the Alzheimer's population means facing tripling the current costs—$300 billion a year, and without a cure in sight.

Why Should You Care, if You Don't Have Alzheimer's Already?

One in ten people over the age of sixty-five will get Alzheimer's disease. By the time you get to age eighty-five, you have an almost fifty-fifty chance. Waiting to play the odds that you will not get Alzheimer's disease is a bad move.

Changes in Super Aging, Normal Aging, and Neurodegenerative Diseases

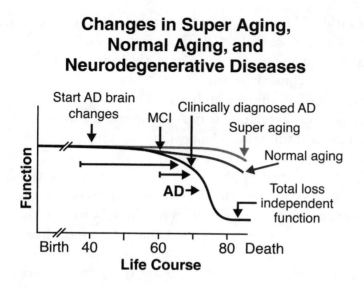

We now know that the brain changes that take place in Alzheimer's disease begin years and even decades before symptoms show, when the plaques, tangles, and amyloid clumps accumulate.

Left unchecked, these changes are followed by the later emergence of the cognitive, functional, and neuropsychiatric (medical term for "bad behavior") symptoms I discussed in chapter 1 and will discuss again in chapter 19.

This differential between the start of the pathology and the onset of Alzheimer's symptoms is especially striking because very recent studies show that a number of people whose brains have high volumes of Alzheimer's pathological changes never develop dementia in their lifetime. In a 2006 study published in *Neurology,* more than one-third of seniors who died dementia-free had enough Alzheimer's-related changes in their brains to meet the National Institute of Aging criteria for "intermediate" or "high" likelihood of getting Alzheimer's. The brains of patients whose neurological health were monitored on a long-term basis were analyzed after they died. Among these elderly individuals, the density of neurofibrillary tangles (discussed in chapter 2) in the memory-storing region of the brain correlated with their scores on memory tests. This was equally true of those who were cognitively normal as well those with MCI. This supports earlier research suggesting that the disease can reach a relatively advanced stage without significant clinical symptoms.

The thrust of all this research is simple. By the time an individual begins to show symptoms of Alzheimer's, the disease has possibly progressed too far to change the outcome. The time to take preventive steps is now. Think of it like this: by the time a person is noticeably affected by the "fallout" of Alzheimer's, the figurative disease "bomb" has already exploded deep within the brain. After that point, current treatments merely seek to treat the symptoms and find ways to offset the damage that has already been done.

Scientists now believe that there are three continuous phases in the neurological development of a person destined to get Alzheimer's. The presymptomatic, or latent, stage lasts for decades. In this stage, Alzheimer's changes to the brain cells accumulate undetected. This may be more likely to occur in individuals who are genetically predisposed to developing Alzheimer's. Interestingly, individuals who eventually develop clinical Alzheimer's (who are followed in research programs that measure memory on an annual or recurring basis) tend to show subtle changes on memory tests years before they manifest symptoms of memory loss or dementia. The record of these subtle changes revealed through testing and brain imaging might lend itself to establishing a means of predicting who will develop Alzheimer's in the future. This is addressed further in chapter 19.

The Challenges to Studying Alzheimer's Prevention

The preventive strategies I will outline in the following chapters are, by scientific standards, premature. They have yet to be thoroughly vetted in randomized clinical trials (drug/intervention versus placebo) to gain the scientific and social acceptance needed for large-scale applications in healthy people. The reason for this is simple. To answer authoritatively on the ifs and hows of prevention—what specific drugs, vitamins, supplements, or interventions could actually prevent Alzheimer's—requires huge studies. Each of these studies represents a major research investment. Another concern is that much of the research community is dominated by a pharmaceutical industry that is far more focused on a cure than on prevention. Finally, to test if these drugs or supplements really prevent Alzheimer's, healthy people have to consider the risks and benefits and be willing to participate in clinical trials.

So far, of the primary prevention strategies already attempted (medications and vitamin studies, discussed in parts 2 and 3), none have shown any benefit for those who have already developed Alzheimer's disease. This may mean that to be effective, potential prevention measures need to be taken long before even the earliest symptoms of dementia emerge. The other possibility is that the agents in question may produce effects too weak to be relevant to the treatment or prevention of Alzheimer's disease. More research is needed to discover which is the case.

From current Alzheimer's prevention studies, it is clear that many challenges must be overcome for such studies to succeed. Some of these challenges include:

- Recruiting enough eligible participants to make data statistically valuable
- Ensuring that the participants are willing to stay in the study for long periods of time and will not drop out
- Having participants who are willing to take the medications prescribed as part of the study
- Designing a study for adequate length to see an effect

If there are not enough participants, then a study is unlikely to show a difference between people getting the real drug and those receiving the placebo. If they don't stay in the study long enough, then the same problem will occur (inability to tell a difference between the real drug and the placebo). Then there is the willingness of research participants to take medications. Many people are reluctant to do so because of the perception of being a guinea pig, or, conversely, concerns that their health will be compromised if they are given only a placebo over a period of time rather than an effective drug. The reality of research is quite different. It is discussed in chapter 20.

Finally, the major issue obstructing primary prevention trials is the cost. Current cost estimates charged to the American taxpayer are $20 to 60 million per drug per study. In fact, pharmaceutical companies spend over 200 million dollars per drug to bring them through the FDA approval process and to the marketplace.

Eat right, exercise daily, and maintain an active lifestyle. This is not exactly new advice on the health front when it comes to preventing heart disease, cancer, and diabetes. But the question I get asked more and more is: "Will doing all these great things prevent me from getting Alzheimer's disease as well?"

There are, in fact, many recent studies suggesting that a combination of diet, exercise, supplements, and healthy habits could delay or prevent Alzheimer's disease. The details are laid out in the rest of this book. Of course, this is not the answer most people are looking for. You would undoubtedly prefer a straight yes or no answer. But the challenge we face as researchers is that attempting to prevent a very complex disease like Alzheimer's is an equally complex undertaking. Since we think a combination of environment, genetics, and other risk factors contributes to the development of this terrible and disabling disease, isolating particular conditions or contributing risks we might prevent is tricky and is complicated further by constant changes that occur over the course of an individual's lifetime.

For example, some studies have shown that an early-life head trauma increases one's risk of developing Alzheimer's later in life. Therefore, a specific event like that is somewhat preventable. Other risk factors for Alzheimer's, such as advancing age, are clearly out of our control.

So can we prevent Alzheimer's? I have three answers for you. Yes, no, and maybe.

Yes, Alzheimer's Is Preventable

If all the recommendations of this book are eventually supported through more and more scientific study, then most Alzheimer's may eventually be preventable. That's because most risk factors can be offset and most interventions are fairly simple.

Among the potential dementia-fighting weapons researchers are looking into are cognitively demanding activities, physical exercise, diet, vitamins and certain dietary supplements, hormone therapy, anti-inflammatory drugs, and statins. It may turn out that by incorporating some or all of these into one's daily routine, a person could influence his or her personal likelihood and timeline for getting Alzheimer's disease. All of these are discussed in detail in upcoming chapters.

No, Alzheimer's Is Not Preventable

Some risk for Alzheimer's disease may be inevitable, and we cannot intervene. As things stand now, by the time the disease is present, it is too late to stop the disease; the best we can hope for is to lessen the symptoms and slow the decline. Alternatively, because some risks are unalterable (genetics, heredity, age, gender), some perceive that developing Alzheimer's is inevitable. This view is fundamentally nihilistic and, unfortunately, very pervasive among the general public and even among most doctors who treat elderly patients affected with dementia or Alzheimer's. If that is the point of view of most people, then prevention is not realistic as a target. It would suggest, however, that a large body of scientific evidence should be ignored, and that is not valid, either.

Maybe Alzheimer's Is Preventable

If the data presented in this book, most of which is based on large population-based surveys, are clinically applicable, then we *may be* able to delay or prevent Alzheimer's altogether.

Look at it this way: if someone follows all of the recommendations laid out in this book but still gets Alzheimer's at age

eighty-five, then he or she might say, "Well, these recommendations didn't work." If that person had not followed the recommendations, however, he or she might have gotten Alzheimer's at age
seventy-five. The hard truth is that, right now, there are no clear
answers.

The other piece of *maybe* is that no single recommendation will
probably be sufficient to affect the outcome significantly on its
own, but all the recommendations taken together are likely to be
far more effective. Again, Alzheimer's is a very complex disease,
and potential prevention measures will need to be similarly
complex—a combination approach that addresses multiple aspects
of the disease development.

In fact, there is too much scientific knowledge about Alzheimer's
to ignore. Because we understand its biology, we are able to identify targets for intervention and prevention. Now that we understand the interactions between the heart and the brain, and
between conditions such as diabetes and amyloid, we can develop
real targets of prevention.

Beyond Alzheimer's, though, every recommendation in this
book makes good health sense. As you can see, the costs and challenges of doing prevention studies make them difficult to conduct.
That translates into reluctance by granting agencies to invest in
these studies. While we wait for solid results from clinical trials,
decades may pass. We must also wait for more clinical trials to be
designed and conducted, to pursue new, possible breakthroughs.
During that time, following these recommendations that we
already know are helpful will lead to better overall health—and
may help slow or even stop Alzheimer's along the way.

In summary, primary prevention studies focusing on a wide
spectrum of potential cognitive, pharmacological, and environmental interventions are still in their infancy. Still, when it has
already been shown that some of these preventive strategies are
already supported by a plethora of epidemiological and laboratory
data, you have to ask yourself, Why wait?

Final Thoughts and Recommendations

- Changes in the brain that cause Alzheimer's symptoms start to accumulate *decades* before a person ever displays any symptoms.

- Prevention of Alzheimer's disease is more desirable than a cure because it may mean fewer people are actually contracting the disease altogether.

- With the rapid aging of the population, the cost of Alzheimer's is exploding.

- Clinical trials of drugs that may prevent Alzheimer's are in the pipeline but still in their infancy. Getting a final answer on whether certain drugs, vitamins, supplements, or compounds could prevent Alzheimer's disease will take years.

- The time to begin prevention strategies is now. Prevention starts with *you*.

- Something *can* be done to prevent Alzheimer's.

PART II

Real Risks

4

Your Alzheimer's IQ:
Know Your Risk

There are clearly identifiable risk factors for the development of Alzheimer's. Some of these may be modifiable and others may not. Recognizing the risks is the first step toward matching them to activities that may intervene to change their outcomes.

This chapter has two parts. First, the risks are outlined and keyed to the chapter that hosts their discussion. Then we take a look at the blood tests that can be used to screen for the particular risk of cognitive decline.

Risk Factors for Cognitive Decline and Alzheimer's

Unmodifiable

Age (this chapter)

Genetic influences, such as heredity and family history (this chapter)

APOE status (this chapter)

Female gender (this chapter)

Modifiable

Hypertension (high blood pressure) (chapter 9)

Elevated cholesterol (chapter 13)

High homocysteine levels (this chapter)

Diabetes-elevated insulin levels (and the metabolic syndrome) (chapter 5)

Heart disease (chapter 7)

Cerebrovascular disease (strokes and transient ischemic attacks [TIAs]) (chapter 7)

Head injury (chapter 8)

Environmental exposure to toxins (chapter 8)

Deficiency of folic acid vitamin (this chapter and chapter 17)

Obesity, especially during midlife (chapter 6)

Risk Factors

In this section, I give an overview of risk factors that are not modifiable. Thankfully, the number of modifiable risk factors surpasses them. Each modifiable risk factor is described in more detail in other chapters throughout the book, as noted previously.

Age

Alzheimer's is a disease of aging. Thus, advanced age is the strongest risk factor for Alzheimer's; risk increases exponentially with age. In other words, the older you live, the higher the risk. As discussed in the previous chapter, at age sixty-five, 5 percent of people have it. That risk doubles with every five years of age. Some estimate that the risk is as high as 50 percent by age eighty-five, but most experts have settled on 35 to 40 percent after age eighty-five. Given the fact that the sixty-five-year-old segment of our population is growing at a faster rate than are any of the others, and that more than 34 million Americans are sixty-five or older, this puts that age range squarely at risk.

Unfortunately, this risk never goes away. Thus, you can never outlive some risk of getting Alzheimer's disease. On the other hand, you can potentially reach the end of your life without ever experiencing symptoms of the disease. In Sun City, at our research institute, we see clients day in and day out who are from their mideighties through a hundred years old, yet who are completely normal from a memory standpoint. These elderly are part of our brain donation/body donation program, so we see them regularly, and, when they pass on, we have had their permission to perform autopsies on them in the interest of medical research. In these individuals, we see very mild Alzheimer's changes within their brains, but none are demented. In fact, by the age of ninety, more than 90 percent of Sun City's cognitively normal elderly experience no Alzheimer's changes in their brains.

Genetic Influences: Heredity and Family History

We can't choose our parents and we can't choose their genetics. Genes and other biological markers are rapidly being identified, which can provide estimates of risk to individuals for the eventual development of complex late-onset diseases such as Alzheimer's, years before symptoms appear. Nevertheless, we still have a poor understanding of genetic influences on cognitive and emotional health.

Although greater than 95 percent of Alzheimer's is considered to be *multifactorial* (meaning attributable to several causes) in terms of etiology (the study of causes of illness), three genes—amyloid precursor protein, presenilin I, and presenilin II—have been identified, in which one or more mutations nearly always result in onset of Alzheimer's before age sixty-five *and* the pattern of inheritance is clearly identified. Alzheimer's disease from these three genetic mutations run in families. These mutations are quite rare but account for many cases of the Alzheimer's seen in the younger age groups (ages thirty-five through sixty). A form of this kind of Alzheimer's was showcased in the touching documentary *The Forgetting* by Dale Shenk, broadcast on PBS in 2002.

A blood test that can identify people with some forms of genetically transmitted Alzheimer's is commercially available. Unfortunately, all the test can do is determine whether someone is at risk;

the mutation is nonetheless likely to be passed on to future generations. Some of the other presenilin tests are not commercially available.

One Family's History

A few years ago, John, a forty-one-year-old gentleman, came to see me. It was clear from my assessment that he was developing Alzheimer's disease. He had lost his job because he was having trouble completing work-related tasks; it emerged that he had been having trouble as early as age thirty-eight or thirty-nine. What tipped me off to concerns about this being Alzheimer's disease was the fact that he had a forty-two-year-old brother who had been diagnosed with Alzheimer's, as well as a mother who had died in her sixties and who had had memory loss. His presentation was alarming given his young age and family history. I was able to confer with his brother's doctor, order the presenillin test, and confirm the diagnosis with a PET scan (chapter 19). What was particularly sad about this case was that he had three children. I referred the family to a genetic counselor. Since that time, he has been placed in a care facility.

The apolipoprotein E (APO-E) gene is associated with a higher risk of both familial and sporadic forms of late-onset Alzheimer's. The APO-E gene is neither necessary nor sufficient to cause the disease and therefore is considered a genetic risk factor or genetic susceptibility gene, rather than an outright cause of Alzheimer's. It is discussed in detail later in this chapter.

Family History

Often I am asked as a clinician to explain the risk of one's developing Alzheimer's if a family member has it. Many family members of patients with Alzheimer's are increasingly aware of and concerned with their own or their offspring's risk of inheriting the disease. Sometimes, brothers, sisters, sons, and daughters of people with Alzheimer's may dismiss concerns about their own risk as unseemly while the family member who actually has Alzheimer's is living. Nevertheless, I have found that many relatives are deeply worried about their own likelihood of developing Alzheimer's and want to understand that possibility more fully.

They may well have reason to be concerned: the additional risk for developing dementia among first-degree relatives of demented people (that is, a mother, father, sister, or brother related by blood has developed Alzheimer's) compared with cognitively normal elderly subjects without a family history of the disease may be up to six times higher. The MIRAGE Study, a national multicenter study from Boston University, run by my colleague Dr. Lindsay Farrer, looks at genetic risk factors influencing the development of Alzheimer's (we are a participating site at SHRI). This study has documented a cumulative risk of developing Alzheimer's among first-degree relatives of about double the incidence (meaning twice as likely) as the risk in nonrelatives. Unaffected brothers and sisters of Alzheimer's patients have a two- to fourfold increased risk of developing dementia, above that of the age-equivalent general population.

Other researchers in Washington, D.C., and New York have demonstrated that the manifestation of Alzheimer's in a first-degree relative increases the lifetime risk of Alzheimer's for an individual by threefold. Although other, nongenetic factors, such as head injury and a low level of education, have also been associated with a higher risk of Alzheimer's, none of these has been as consistent as a family history in identifying individuals at risk.

Female Gender

Although Alzheimer's is not selective in who is afflicted, we know that women have a higher risk of developing Alzheimer's. In individuals older than sixty-five, Alzheimer's affects roughly two to three times more women than men. Overall, the ratio is 60:40

women to men. This may be related to a survival differential, as men have a shorter life expectancy (by three to five years). However, it may also be related to estrogen exposure. This is discussed in more detail in chapter 10.

The gender difference in Alzheimer's is a consistent finding. There has been significant focus on estrogen as related to Alzheimer's. A community-based study of a Stockholm population of 1,500 women has shown that incidence of Alzheimer's continues to increase with age, but only among women after the age of seventy-nine. In this group, older women have a higher incidence. In that particular study, simply being a woman tripled the relative risk of Alzheimer's. Preliminary data from the Stockholm study suggest that early menopause may also represent a risk factor of incidence in women. Similar results have been reported from other epidemiological studies in the United Kingdom and the Netherlands. In addition, women with a history of myocardial infarction are five times more likely to develop Alzheimer's than are those without such a history.

So the question is, why do women get Alzheimer's disease more often than do men? One possibility is that estrogen may be lost in the brains of women with Alzheimer's disease. In a recently announced study from the Sun Health Research Institute and the University of Chicago, analysis of women who had died with Alzheimer's disease showed that their brains had much less estrogen content than the brains of women who were age-matched controls. This estrogen loss might explain why there is a higher prevalence of Alzheimer's disease in women than in men. Animal experiments have shown that estrogen deficiency accelerates amyloid production and deposition. Indeed, estrogen depletion leads to a decline of declarative memory and motor coordination, which may be prevented by estrogen therapy. Some of these findings are explained further in chapter 10.

When estrogen has been looked at in the blood, however, these findings were not supported, suggesting that this is a phenomenon unique to the brain. Serum (blood) estrogen was low in normal elderly women and in those with Alzheimer's. As my colleague Dr. Rena Li suggests, brain estrogen deficiency is more specific than blood estrogen deficiency in the development of Alzheimer's disease.

Another consequence of reduced estrogen might relate to how changes in the brain occur in Alzheimer's. It has been discovered that plaques and tangles (discussed in chapter 2) are much more powerfully associated with Alzheimer's in women than in men. A study of nuns and priests found that the more plaques and tangles found in the brain, the higher the probability of clinical Alzheimer's in women as compared with men. These data add to the growing evidence that women are more vulnerable than men are to developing Alzheimer's.

Need-to-Know Blood Test Values

Some of the risks for getting Alzheimer's are identifiable by blood tests; others are not. While routine blood tests can reveal some of these risks, others require special panels above and beyond a regular blood test. The test results vary, some of them indicating unique factors that point to risk of Alzheimer's disease and others indicating only the presence of physiological abnormalities that may or may not represent the risk of Alzheimer's.

Homocysteine

One of the numbers you should know is for a blood protein called *homocysteine*. Homocysteine is identified through a simple blood test that any physician can order. High homocysteine levels in the blood go hand in hand with folic acid (a B vitamin) deficiency, and have been associated with higher rates of Alzheimer's disease, vascular dementia, heart disease, and stroke.

Homocysteine levels are already frequently monitored by neurologists and cardiologists, who have been aware for a long time of a well-established link between elevated homocysteine levels—known as *hyperhomocysteinemia*—and cardiovascular and *ischemic* (reduced oxygen and nutrients to the brain) events. For example, elevated homocysteine levels have long been recognized as a significant risk factor for stroke. In the last several years, scientists have found links between elevated homocysteine levels and higher risk of Alzheimer's disease, in prospective population-based studies.

The link between elevated homocysteine levels and Alzheimer's was first seen in the famous Framingham study, an ongoing project that has investigated the risk of heart disease and other diseases in residents of Framingham, Massachusetts, for the past thirty years through regular medical evaluations. In a recent population-based study in Italy, researchers found that elevated plasma homocysteine levels effectively doubled individuals' risk of developing dementia, as did folate deficiencies.

Other studies published recently revealed that hyperhomocysteinemia not only increases your risk for Alzheimer's disease but is often found coupled with more mild declines in cognitive function and memory. Scientists from the Baltimore Memory Study found that elevated levels of homocysteine were strongly and consistently linked to poorer performance on memory and other cognitive tests, compared with the scores of individuals with normal-range homocysteine levels. This was true in all eight parts of the memory tests. Subjects in the highest quartile (meaning the top 25 percent) of homocysteine levels were two times more likely to be in the lowest quarterile on cognitive test scores than those in the lowest quartile of homocysteine levels—and the dementia risk between these two quartiles was equal to four years tacked on to the lives of those with hyperhomocysteinemia. This is a significant difference and is important in understanding Alzheimer's because homocysteine is one risk factor that we *can* do something about.

So, what exactly is homocysteine and what is its link to Alzheimer's disease? Homocysteine is a *sulfhydryl*-containing amino acid, which means that it is a building block of a protein made naturally in the body. Homocysteine is a derivative of the essential amino acid *methionine*, which is abundant in proteins. In the body, the conversion of methionine to homocysteine is crucial to the proper functioning of a host of biomolecules that include DNA, neurotransmitters, phospholipids, and proteins.

Scientists know that homocysteine is toxic to brain cells (neurons) because it promotes production of free radicals and stimulates glutamatergic activity. When the amount of homocysteine in the bloodstream gets too high, it inhibits DNA repair and makes the DNA strands vulnerable to the toxic effects of amyloid (see chapter 1).

In mice genetically engineered to develop Alzheimer's, a deficiency of folic acid also increased DNA damage and promoted amyloid accumulation. In these models, the elevated homocysteine levels associated with folic acid deficiency inhibit DNA repair in brain cells responsible for memory (the hippocampal neurons). These brain cells are then vulnerable to amyloid toxicity (see chapter 2).

Blood concentrations of homocysteine vary widely, but the concentration of homocysteine inside cells is maintained within a relatively narrow range. Significant increases outside this range can spike risk of heart attack and stroke. In fact, I've actually seen a twenty-four-year-old suffer a major stroke caused by hyperhomocysteinemia.

Increased levels of homocysteine in the plasma have been investigated vigorously as a modifiable cause for development of stroke and heart disease. Elevations in homocysteine can be caused by genetic mutations, age, vitamin deficiencies, diseases, and other lifestyle factors, including excessive alcohol, coffee, tobacco consumption, or physical inactivity. Diseases that can result in a vitamin deficiency can also raise homocysteine levels. Some of these include pernicious anemia (low blood counts of red blood cells), severe kidney disease or renal failure, low thyroid levels (called *hypothyroidism* by medical personnel; explained in more detail in the following section), diabetes, psoriasis, and cancer. Medications, including lipid-lowering drugs for cholesterol, arthritis medication, anticonvulsants (for epilepsy), sex hormones, and other chemicals can increase homocysteine, too.

Here's what you need to know about measuring your homocysteine level:

- It is a simple blood test.

- The normal range is 4 to 12 micromol/L.
- Mildly elevated levels are 13 to 20 micromol/L.
- Severely elevated levels are above 20 micromol/dl.

Thyroid Functions

Low thyroid function (called hypothyroidism) is a well-known cause of memory loss and dementia. Thyroid failure or severe hypothyroidism is characterized by high blood levels of *thyroid-stimulating hormone* (a hormone from the brain that stimulates thyroid hormone production, also known as TSH), and reduced levels of thyroid hormones thyroxine and triiodothyronine (called T3 and T4, respectively) in the blood. Hypothyroidism, characterized by the failure of the thyroid gland to clear iodine from the body, is found in some elderly patients.

Hypothyroidism can cause dementia independent of Alzheimer's. This dementia is often associated with mental changes, including depression, poor concentration, and attention problems. Other characteristics of hypothyroidism include sensitivity to cold; constipation; pale dry skin; puffy face; hoarse voice; unexplained weight gain; muscle aches; muscle tenderness and stiffness; pain, stiffness, or swelling in joints; muscle weakness; fatigue; and lethargy. Hypothyroidism has also been implicated as possibly contributing to Alzheimer's disease.

Your levels of thyroid function are pretty easy to ascertain because T3, T4, and TSH levels are monitored regularly in medical practice. Ask your physician if you are unsure of when your thyroid was last checked.

Here is what you need to know about testing for thyroid functions:

- It is a simple blood test.
- The normal range for TSH is 0.4 to 4.0mIU/L.
- The normal range for T4 is 4.5 to 11.2mcg/dl.
- The normal range for T3 is 0.1 to 0.2 mcg/dl.

Diabetes

Diabetes, especially type 2 diabetes, is a big risk factor for Alzheimer's disease. The insulin resistance that characterizes type 2 diabetes is also believed to precipitate Alzheimer's pathology through inflammatory changes in the brain. But recent studies show that a class of diabetes drug, thiazolidinediones, may wield a powerful protective effect against developing dementia, and diabetes, caught early, is a highly manageable disease. As part of your Alzheimer's risk IQ, get your insulin levels, blood sugar, and hemoglobin A1C, which may indicate diabetes, checked by your physician. I'll discuss the link between diabetes and Alzheimer's at greater length in the next chapter.

Here's what you need to know about testing for diabetes:

- It involves blood tests and a glucose tolerance test.
- The normal range for blood sugar is 70 to 100 mg/dl. Blood sugars should be checked after fasting for twelve hours.
- Another test is the glucose tolerance test. This involves drinking a sugary liquid and having your blood sugars tested every hour for three hours.
- Another blood test checks your glycosolated hemoglobin (HbA1C). The normal range is less than 5 percent. Mildly elevated is 5 to 7.0 percent, and significantly elevated is greater than 7 percent.
- Another blood test measures your fasting insulin levels. The normal range is less than 25 microU/ml.

Apolipoprotein E Genotype

Recent advances in genetic research on Alzheimer's have brought about the possibility of genetic susceptibility testing for asymptomatic individuals. The Apolipoprotein E genotype, which can be determined by a blood test, can identify one of the most powerful risk factors. This test simply tells which of three *apolipoprotein E* types (alleles) we have in our blood: APO-Eε2, APO-Eε3, and APO-Eε4.

Apolipoproteins are blood proteins that carry fat and choles-terol in the blood to and from the liver. There are many types of apolipoproteins. All of them are derived from the genes you inher-ited from your mother and father.

The APO-E blood test is commercially available through a company called Athena Diagnostics (www.athenadiagnostics.com) and costs $315. There may be other ways to get the blood test, but ask your doctor or go to a dementia specialist. Be aware that this test is usually not covered by Medicare, and coverage by individ-ual insurance plans varies.

Research indicates that an APO-Eε2 genotype, which is quite rare, might provide some protection against Alzheimer's. APO-Eε3 is the most common form and is neutral in terms of Alzheimer's risk. The APO-Eε4 genotype, less common than APO-Eε3, is found in about half the people with Alzheimer's disease and is present in one-fifth of people with no Alzheimer's disease.

APO-E is a blood type like A, B, and O are blood types. Like all other blood types, APO-E is inherited with one copy of the gene from your mother and another copy of the gene from your father. Studies have shown that if you have two copies of the APO-Eε4, your risk for the development or Alzheimer's disease is thirteen times that of the general population. If you have one copy of the APO-Eε4, your risk is three to four times greater than it is for the general population. This is depicted in the figure on page 73. The bars on the right show the increased chance of developing Alzheimer's associated with being an APO-Eε4 carrier.

So the APO-E genotype blood test becomes a very powerful way of identifying people who are at risk for Alzheimer's. That is both the good news and the bad news—the latter being, is it bad to know if you are a carrier of this blood type?

My colleague Dr. Robert Green, at Boston University Medical School, aims to find out. Dr. Green is leading a study called the Risk Evaluation and Education for Alzheimer's (REVEAL), the first randomized controlled trial (RCT) of its kind to evaluate the impact of Alzheimer's risk assessment using APO-E genotype disclosure.

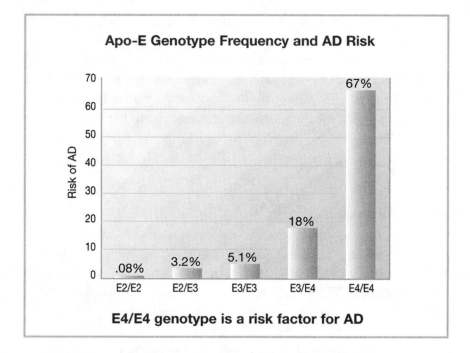

APO-E genotype frequency and Alzheimer's risk.

In the REVEAL study, the investigators contact at-risk people to determine if they wish to be evaluated and notified of their genetic risk for developing the disease. All study participants are adult children of someone with clinically diagnosed and/or autopsy-confirmed Alzheimer's. The major questions in this portion of the study include who seeks this information and why.

So far, the people seeking this information tend to be younger than age sixty, college educated, and female. The main reasons participants have given for wanting to know their genotype include:

- To contribute to research (93.9 percent)
- To arrange personal affairs (87.4 percent)
- In hope that effective treatment will be developed (86.8 percent)

But the best predictor of why people actually pursued getting the blood test was the need to prepare family members for Alzheimer's. In fact, participants endorsed this reason three times more than they did other reasons. Early findings from REVEAL suggest that genetic susceptibility testing is of interest to at-risk individuals, even in the relative absence of available treatments.

CASE STUDY

Getting a Blood Test

Brian, a retired educator in his mid- to late sixties, came to see me some years ago, expressing concern that he might be in line for Alzheimer's disease. His mother had Alzheimer's and was still alive. He wished to learn from me how much risk he had for developing Alzheimer's himself and wanted to undergo "the blood test" for Alzheimer's.

I told him the reality that because his mother had a diagnosed case of Alzheimer's disease, his chances were two- to threefold. We discussed using the APO-E genotype as a way of identifying his risk, but I counseled him that this test was not routinely used to screen asymptomatic people (those without memory loss before they manifest any symptoms), and that both the American Medical Association and the American Academy of Neurology had both recommended against routine screening. Nevertheless, he decided he wanted to have the test done. His results came back 4–4 (two copies of APO-Eε4), which put him at a tremendous risk—about thirteen times the normal risk for getting Alzheimer's. The gentleman took this information well and used it as a motivator to engage in health habits I've underscored in this book. Since implementing an aggressive preventive therapy strategy four years ago, he continues to show no Alzheimer's symptoms.

So what does it mean if you have an ε4? Does that mean that you are going to get Alzheimer's disease? Not necessarily. To begin with, having this gene does not necessarily mean that a person will develop this disease; it only indicates that the person is at greater risk to do so. There are people with the ε4 gene who go to their graves having never experiencing Alzheimer's. Conversely, many people who develop Alzheimer's disease do not have even one copy of the APO-Eε4 gene—about half of all Alzheimer's patients.

If you have no memory loss (in other words, you are asymptomatic), then you should not be tested routinely because of the potential for discrimination for insurability. The way to get around this includes having your parents (especially if one or the other is affected by Alzheimer's) tested to determine your risk indirectly. If you do have symptoms, I recommend getting the test but only under the supervision of someone who has experience in this area and can counsel you accordingly.

If you have memory loss and you are an ε4 carrier, however, the chance that some of your memory loss may be related to Alzheimer's disease is tremendously high. My colleague Dr. Norman Relkin, of Weill Cornell Medical College in New York, estimates it at about 94 to 97 percent. And we know that people with pre-Alzheimer's mild cognitive impairment (MCI) are much more likely to progress to full Alzheimer's disease if they are carriers of ε4 than are people who do not have the ε4 gene. Among ε4 carriers with mild cognitive impairment, 50 percent converted from MCI to Alzheimer's within three years, compared with noncarriers, of whom only 20 percent converted over the same time period. Interestingly, MCI individuals with the ε4 gene seem to respond better to memory medication such as donepezil (Aricept) than do mild cognitively impaired individuals without an ε4.

In multiple studies, an increased frequency of the APO-Eε4 allele has been associated with the worsening cognitive function. My colleague Dr. Richard Caselli, of the Mayo Clinic in Scottsdale, found that age-related memory impairment occurred earlier in people aged forty-nine to sixty-nine years old who had a double copy of APO-Eε4, compared with memory loss in those lacking APO-Eε4. In a different study, researchers found that the metabolic changes that take place in an Alzheimer's brain were detectable by positron emission tomography (PET) scans in even younger adult carriers of ε4 (twenty- to forty-year-olds). PET scans are explained in more detail in chapter 20. However, a study in Korea found no association of ε4 carrier status with performance on neuropsychological tests. In the Religious Orders Study from Chicago, researchers found a strong association between APO-Eε4 and impaired cognitive function immediately before death. The ε4 allele was associated with a twofold increased risk for cognitive decline among nearly one thousand subjects over the seven-year longitudinal MacArthur Study of Successful Aging. Together, these studies indicate that carrying an APO-Eε4 not only increases one's risk for Alzheimer's but could also affect cognitive function before the disease takes hold.

How common is it to see ε4 with MCI? Study results vary, but current estimates indicate that between 30 and 50 percent of people with diagnosed MCI have an ε4. Remember, 20 percent of the nondemented general population and up to half of people with Alzheimer's have an ε4.

Interestingly, the frequency of ε4 varies by location in the world, even from country to country. In Greece, only 8 percent of people have the ε4, whereas in Sweden, the Netherlands, and England, between 26 and 34 percent of the general population have it. Such genetic heterogeneity in different populations around the world may account for the variant incidences of Alzheimer's disease worldwide.

Myths and Truths about APO-E Genotyping

Myth: If I have an ε4, I will get Alzheimer's for sure.

Not true: Having an ε4 merely increases the risk of getting Alzheimer's.

Myth: If I don't have an ε4, I will not get Alzheimer's.

Not true: Up to 50 percent of people with Alzheimer's do not have an ε4.

Myth: I can change the presence or absence of having an ε4.

Not true: Your APO-E status is in your genetic makeup from the moment of conception.

Myth: If neither of my parents has an ε4, I cannot inherit it.

True: One of your parents must carry an ε4 for you to inherit one. If a parent has a double copy, then he or she has passed it on to you. If he or she has one copy, there is a fifty-fifty chance of inheriting it.

CASE STUDY

Getting a Genetic Test

Steve, a retired police officer, came to seem me first when he was fifty-seven years old. He had worked in Chicago as a highly decorated detective but had retired to Las Vegas.

Within a few years, he started having trouble with his memory, manifested in difficulty completing projects around the house. After a series of evaluations, he was diagnosed with Alzheimer's. A genetic test revealed that he had a double copy of the APO-Eε4 allele (4–4). Like many with this genetic profile, he manifested a particularly aggressive case of Alzheimer's. Although he fought the disease with the best and most current treatments and in the most dignified manner, he died tragically at the incredibly young age of fifty-nine. His passing was felt by many who knew him.

Cholesterol-Lipid Panel

Elevated cholesterol may also be a risk factor for Alzheimer's. As a person transitions from normal cognitive function to the pre-Alzheimer's condition of mild cognitive impairment, his or her blood cholesterol level goes up. Luckily, many doctors devote their careers to treating cholesterol for reasons that have more to do with heart disease than Alzheimer's, so the chances are you have already undergone the simple blood test that gives you a breakdown of your cholesterol levels. The basic strategy is to lower your LDL, lower your total cholesterol (TC), lower your triglycerides, and elevate your HDL. Another goal is to improve the TC/HDL ratio; the higher one's TC/HDL ratio, the higher one's risk for developing heart attacks.

The National Cholesterol Educational Panel (NCEP) sets the standard cholesterol targets for individuals as indicating their risk for heart disease, family history, and diabetes. The NCEP has not yet taken up recommendations for individuals with Alzheimer's but one might easily appropriate their guidelines for our preventive strategies. The lipid panel has many parts to it:

- HDL (high-density lipoprotein, aka "good cholesterol")
- LDL (low-density lipoprotein, aka "bad cholesterol")
- VLDL (very low-density lipoprotein, aka "very bad cholesterol")
- Total cholesterol (HDL + LDL + VLDL = TC)
- Cholesterol ratio (total cholesterol/ HDL)
- Triglycerides (aka fat or lipids)

What is the normal range for total cholesterol?
Less than 199 mg/dl is desirable, 200 to 239 mg/dl is borderline, and more than 240 mg/dl is considered high risk

What is the normal range for LDL?
Less than 100 mg/dl is optimal, 100 to 129 mg/dl is near/above optimal, 130 to 159 mg/dl is borderline high, 160 to 189 mg/dl is considered high, and more than 189 mg/dl is considered very high.

What is the normal range for triglycerides?
Less than 150 mg/dl is normal, 150 to 199 mg/dl is borderline high, 200 to 499 mg/dl is high, and more than 499 mg/dl is considered very high.

What is the normal range for the cholesterol ratio?
The lower, the better. For men, optimal is less than 3.5 and for women, less than 3.3. The average ratio for men is 5.0, and 4.4 for women. Increased risk is 5.0 for men and 4.5 for women.

Cholesterol levels should be checked while fasting. Ask your doctor if the values listed here are right for you.

My colleague Dr. Larry Sparks (who has spent his whole career exploring the link between cholesterol and Alzheimer's) at Sun Health Research Institute has worked to compare elevated cholesterol levels with brain function. He took blood samples from individuals enrolled in our brain and body donation program and then measured both the cholesterol levels and the appearance of amyloid in brain tissue of patients who, at the time of their deaths, were cognitively normal, had mild cognitive impairment, or suffered from full-blown Alzheimer's.

What Dr. Sparks found was that the cholesterol level rises progressively as an individual transitions from normal cognitive function to Alzheimer's, but does not change once a person has Alzheimer's. This suggests that cholesterol is involved in the primary cascade of Alzheimer's changes in the brain and supports the larger view that cholesterol control should be addressed in any thorough Alzheimer's prevention plan. We will discuss this more in chapter 13.

Final Thoughts and Recommendations

- There are clear risk factors for developing Alzheimer's; some are modifiable and some are not.
- Unmodifiable risk factors include age, family history, genetic influences, and being of the female gender.
- Modifiable risk factors include hypertension, cholesterol, heart disease, obesity, cerebrovascular disease, head injury, vitamin deficiency, diabetes, and elevated homocysteine levels.
- Have your doctor monitor your thyroid levels.
- Have your doctor monitor your vitamin B_{12} and folic acid levels.
- Have your doctor periodically check your homocysteine level.

- Have your doctor check you for diabetes and insulin resistance.
- Consider getting tested for the Apolipoprotein E genotype, if you strongly suspect that this may be a factor.
- Have your doctor monitor your cholesterol.

5

Diabetes

The number of cases of type 2 diabetes has been on a meteoric rise in the United States and abroad. The World Health Organization puts the number of people who have diabetes worldwide at 177 million, and the figure is likely to reach 300 million by the year 2025. In the United States, someone is diagnosed with diabetes every sixty seconds, according to the American Diabetes Association, adding to the 18 million current patients nationwide and an estimated 9 million more that remain undiagnosed. One reason for the proliferation of diabetes is related to the bulging American waistline.

So what does this have to do with Alzheimer's disease? The answer, scientists are discovering, seems to be "A great deal." Links between abnormal insulin regulation or insulin resistance, both precursors of type 2 diabetes, and a person's risk of Alzheimer's disease have been borne out in numerous epidemiological and clinical studies.

But back to basics: What is diabetes? Who has it? And how could it affect your risk of getting Alzheimer's?

A Definition

Diabetes is a condition whereby a person's body either loses its ability to properly produce insulin or ignores the insulin it makes. Although this classification is simplified for the purposes of this discussion, diabetes is generally subdivided into two categories, type 1 and type 2. Type 1 occurs when the body does not produce enough insulin (a hormone made by the pancreas). As a result of this deficiency, the body cannot metabolize sugar in the blood, and therefore cells can starve from lack of sugar (which is essential for energy production). Type 1 diabetes tends to be diagnosed in childhood, adolescence, or young adulthood when unmistakable symptoms indicate the condition. It is usually treated with injected insulin, but now there are alternative routes for administering that insulin, including as a nasal spray and via an implanted pump. Type 1 diabetics must monitor their blood sugars daily to ensure that their blood sugars do not get too high or too low, as both extremes can be quite dangerous. Type 1 diabetes is not associated with a risk for Alzheimer's disease.

Type 2 diabetes is a condition whereby the cells themselves resist the entry of blood sugar, even when there is adequate insulin in the blood. Type 2 is the most common form of diabetes and is the primary culprit when we turn our attention to the risk of dementia and Alzheimer's.

Diabetes is a disabling condition that can do severe damage to internal organs, particularly the kidneys, the eyes (especially the retinas), and the nerves. It is a leading cause of heart disease, stroke, and kidney failure. Left untreated, it can also lead to lifelong debilitation in the form of dialysis placement, kidney failure, limb loss, and acquired blindness. In a condition called diabetic peripheral neuropathy, the nerves in the feet are damaged, causing a lack of balance or a persistent burning sensation.

Your Brain on Insulin

That there is a link between diabetes, which affects insulin levels in the body, and cognitive function, which relies on insulin in the brain, makes perfect medical sense. Your brain needs a near-constant supply of glucose (blood sugar) to keep going, and insulin is a key player in providing and regulating that nutrient to the brain. Insulin is also responsible for regulating a great deal of activity in the brain cells themselves, as well as acting in the conveyance of signals from one neuron to the next. Because insulin is constantly transported across the blood/brain barrier, the levels of insulin found in the rest of the body tend to correlate with the levels found in the brain. It follows then, that when insulin and glucose metabolism are impaired, cognitive function suffers. Because of this close connection, any disruption in the metabolism of insulin in the rest of the body leading to elevated blood insulin levels (*hyperinsulinemia*) can negatively impact memory, as well as increase the risk of developing Alzheimer's. Interestingly, we can measure metabolic changes related to glucose metabolism in peoples' brains, using PET scans. PET scans are discussed in more detail in chapter 19.

What We Know

Just a decade ago, type 2 diabetes and Alzheimer's were considered to be mutually exclusive. That is, it was unusual to have both. Some small-population studies found neutral or lower risk between type 2 patients and the onset of Alzheimer's. However, more recent studies, using different criteria to determine the presence of diabetes and relying on a more comprehensive analysis of glucose insulin levels, have consistently found an increased risk of Alzheimer's disease in people with type 2 diabetes. In these later studies, a person with diabetes mellitus has about twice the risk of developing Alzheimer's as did a nondiabetic, when controlled for age, education, and other variables. If the person is a woman and/or has the APO-E gene, then the risk is even higher.

Epidemiological studies have shown strong links between the risk of dementia as well as the rate of cognitive decline and an individual's history of diabetes and insulin resistance. One study has indicated that up to 43 percent of dementia could be attributable to diabetes mellitus or stroke, or a combination of the two.

Another study from the Karolinska Institute in Stockholm, Sweden, found that patients with borderline diabetes (defined in chapter 4), aged seventy-five or older, had a 77 percent increased risk of developing Alzheimer's in a nine-year time span, compared with patients who had normal blood sugar levels. The authors attributed this to "impaired insulin processing." Another study, from the Kaiser Permanante Group of Northern California, correlated high levels of glycosolated hemoglobin (HbA1C; see chapter 4) to a risk of developing Alzheimer's. Patients with a very high HbA1C (greater than 15 percent) had a 78 percent greater risk of developing Alzheimer's disease or cognitive decline in the next ten years. Patients with mild elevations of HbA1C had a 16 to 25 percent elevated risk.

Other research has indicated that high insulin levels, as in type 2 diabetes, may convey a specific risk for the development of Alzheimer's, because both brain amyloid metabolism and insulin metabolism regulation are dependent on the same enzyme—*insulin degrading enzyme* (IDE). Specifically, high levels of insulin can cause inflammation in the central nervous system, thereby preventing the normal breakdown of beta-amyloid, the toxic protein that, as we saw in chapter 2, accumulates in the brain of an individual with Alzheimer's. When there is insulin resistance, IDE does not work as well as it should, which results in lesser breakdown of beta-amyloid.

What We Are Still Learning

While these links between diabetes and the onset of Alzheimer's disease can be shown, researchers are still unsure of what they mean. How much does the pathology of insulin disorders translate into a risk for Alzheimer's disease? Or, put another way, could Alzheimer's disease actually be a form of diabetes? That is the tantalizing suggestion from a study recently published in the *Journal of Alzheimer's Disease*. The study showed that insulin production declines early and significantly as Alzheimer's disease advances.

What is so surprising about this discovery is that, until very recently, we didn't know that insulin was produced in the brain at all. We thought all insulin was produced in the pancreas. However, scientists have also recently discovered that Alzheimer's patients produce less insulin than do their nondemented counterparts, a trend that worsens as the disease progresses. Insulin and its related protein, insulin-related-growth factor 1, has the ability to bind to cellular sectors, creating an insulin resistance situation similar to type 2 diabetes and causing brain cells to starve and possibly die.

Researchers still don't completely understand the complex link between type 2 diabetes and the risk of dementia. As with Alzheimer's disease, the disorders and health conditions found in those with type 2 diabetes are numerous. The challenge for researchers is to tease from this web of symptoms and genetic pre-dispositions causal links so that, down the road, we doctors may offer appropriate treatment to our Alzheimer's patients, or better yet, develop a means of prevention. Recent findings show that the effect of insulin disruption and resistance on memory function is complicated and most likely depends on a combination of other factors, such as an individual's age, genetic makeup, and what stage either the diabetes or the dementia has reached.

But if insulin levels and uptake is as influential in memory func-tion as the data suggests, then antidiabetes drugs, anti-inflamma-tory agents, and dietary modifications may all aid in slowing cognitive decline and, consequently, the risk of Alzheimer's.

A new study showed that a class of diabetes drug called thiazolidinediones—Actos (pioglitazone), Avandia (rosiglitazone), and Avandamet (rosiglitazone and metformin)—may have a special protective effect when it comes to Alzheimer's. In a study of 142,328 veterans being treated for diabetes over six years, those prescribed thiazolidinediones were 19 percent less likely to develop Alzheimer's than were those on insulin therapy. Both rosiglitazone and pioglitazone are actively under investigation in clinical trials as potential treatments for Alzheimer's. The trials so far are encouraging. However, the research with rosiglitazone hangs under a cloud because of concerns about heart complications, although this is hotly debated.

And results from a long-running multicenter clinical trial called Diabetes Control and Complications Trial (DCCT) recently showed that aggressive management through tight glycemic control (keeping blood glucose levels low nutritionally) in the earliest stages of diabetes may prevent cognitive decline later on, as well as reduce progression of diabetes's other damaging symptoms.

The link between type 2 diabetes and Alzheimer's continues to be a central therapeutic target squarely in the sights of the national and international medical community.

What You Can Do

Even though we don't yet know whether type 2 diabetes is a primary culprit or has only a small supporting role in patients who eventually develop Alzheimer's, the body of data we have is good and growing, and this much is clear: First, type 2 diabetes has strong links to both the onset of dementia and the decline in cognitive function in both middle and old age. Second, these links are independent of confounding vascular conditions such as heart disease, hypertension, and stroke.

Because of the great number of associated problems and health risks that come with type 2 diabetes, it is important to have your insulin levels and HbA1C regularly checked by your doctor. As the DCCT study results show, the treatment for diabetes does not increase the risk of cognitive decline, and preventing or managing the disease if you have already been diagnosed will lower your risk of hypertension, heart disease, and stroke. It could very well lower your chance of getting Alzheimer's, too.

Final Thoughts and Recommendations

- Diabetes, particularly type 2, increases risk for Alzheimer's.
- Insulin resistance, a key component of type 2 diabetes, has been found in Alzheimer's-affected brains.
- Have your doctor check you for diabetes.
- If you have diabetes, manage it meticulously: your target blood sugar should be 70 to 110; and your target glycosolated hemoglobin (HbA1c), less than 6.6.

- Diabetic medications are being used as potential treatments for Alzheimer's disease.

- If you are diabetic, have your doctor consider putting you on a thiazolidinediones. These are also known as glitazones (rosiglitazone/Avandia) and (pioglitazone/Actos).

6

Body Weight
and Obesity

Obesity, defined medically as a *body mass index* (BMI) of 30 or more grams per meter of one's height squared, is a national epidemic in the United States and is becoming a worldwide health problem, as well. Being overweight is defined as a BMI of 25 to 30. Being morbidly obese (dangerously overweight) is defined as a BMI greater than 40.

Messages about obesity are everywhere, from the media to the shelves at the grocery store. Despite the widespread awareness about the health woes associated with overeating and an $8-billion-plus diet industry largely fueled by desirable physical proportions, the American waistline continues to increase and our food portion sizes increase, too. Obesity, aside from its aesthetic implications, increases risk for many conditions and diseases, including high blood pressure (hypertension), type 2 diabetes, heart disease, and arthritis.

These other health issues aside, how does obesity relate to Alzheimer's disease?

The Link between Obesity and Alzheimer's

New evidence indicates that obesity may play a significant role in cognitive decline and dementia, including the development of Alzheimer's disease. This link has been demonstrated particularly when obesity first appears in middle age.

Determining Your Body Mass Index

BMI	19	20	21	22	23	24	25	26	27	28	29	30	31	32	33	34	35
Height in inches							Body weight in pounds										
58	91	96	100	105	110	115	119	124	129	134	138	143	148	153	158	162	167
59	94	99	104	109	114	119	124	128	133	138	143	148	153	158	163	168	173
60	97	102	107	112	118	123	128	133	138	143	148	153	158	163	168	174	179
61	100	106	111	116	122	127	132	137	143	148	153	158	164	169	174	180	185
62	104	109	115	120	126	131	136	142	147	153	158	164	169	175	180	186	191
63	107	113	118	124	130	135	141	146	152	158	163	169	175	180	186	191	197
64	110	116	122	128	134	140	145	151	157	163	169	174	180	186	192	197	204
65	114	120	126	132	138	144	150	156	162	168	174	180	186	192	198	204	210
66	118	124	130	136	142	148	155	161	167	173	179	186	192	198	204	210	216
67	121	127	134	140	146	153	159	166	172	178	185	191	198	204	211	217	223
68	125	131	138	144	151	158	164	171	177	184	190	197	203	210	216	223	230
69	128	135	142	149	155	162	169	176	182	189	196	203	209	216	223	230	236
70	132	139	146	153	160	167	174	181	188	195	202	209	216	222	229	236	243
71	136	143	150	157	165	172	179	186	193	200	208	215	222	229	236	243	250
72	140	147	154	162	169	177	184	191	199	206	213	221	228	235	242	250	258
73	144	151	159	166	174	182	189	197	204	212	219	227	235	242	250	257	265
74	148	155	163	171	179	186	194	202	210	218	225	233	241	249	256	264	272
75	152	160	168	176	184	192	200	208	216	224	232	240	248	256	264	272	279
76	156	164	172	180	189	197	205	213	221	230	238	246	254	263	271	279	287

The body mass index (BMI) is a fairly accurate way of determining whether you are overweight. Use your finger to find your height and then follow the line to the right to find your weight. Next, move your finger up to the top line (BMI). If your BMI is higher than 25, you are overweight. If your BMI is higher than 30, you are obese.

One of the seminal studies on obesity and Alzheimer's comes out of Finland. There researchers evaluated almost 1,500 people over a span of twenty years, measuring participants' BMI as well as cholesterol levels, blood pressure, height, and weight. The subjects were divided into three groups: those with a normal BMI (less than 25), those who were overweight (a BMI between 25 and 30), and those who had a BMI greater than 30.

The researchers found that obesity in midlife increased the risk for the development of dementia and Alzheimer's disease later in life. Those who were obese in midlife were more than twice as likely to develop Alzheimer's disease later, even when smokers or those who suffered from high blood pressure or high cholesterol were not included in the group. When obesity was *added* to the profile of those who had both high cholesterol and high blood pressure, the risk of developing Alzheimer's increased up to sixfold, suggesting that, added together, these risks were highly predictive of whether or not the person would contract Alzheimer's.

Another study confirmed the link between midlife obesity and dementia risk. Researchers at the University of Washington evaluated five-year data on 3,602 participants from the Cardiovascular Health Cognition Study, a substudy of the Cardiovascular Health Study. During that time, 480 participants received a diagnosis of dementia. The researchers measured the participants' weight and height at the time of their admission into the substudy, to calculate their present BMI. To estimate their midlife BMI, participants were asked to self-report what they thought their weight had been at age fifty. A BMI of 20 kg/m^2 to 25 kg/m^2 was considered normal, while underweight was defined as a BMI of less than 20 kg/m^2, overweight as a BMI of 26 kg/m^2 to 30 kg/m^2, and obese as a BMI of greater than 30 kg/m^2. Researchers took into consideration such factors as age, race, sex, and education, as well as cardiovascular and dementia risk factors. All things considered, the study concluded that being obese at the age of fifty was significantly associated with a 40 percent increased risk of dementia.

Another study done in Sweden showed that higher BMI among women was associated with a particularly high increased risk for dementia. In the Honolulu-Asia aging study, a higher BMI was associated with the risk of vascular dementia (dementia related to strokes; see chapter 1) and other types of dementia in men, but not for Alzheimer's disease.

These findings appear to hold true in the population at large. One study of MRI brain scans found that people who were obese as measured by a higher waist–hip ratio, had a smaller hippocampus, the portion of the brain responsible for memory, than did those with lower waist–hip ratios. This suggests that obesity might accelerate neurological degeneration or blood vessel changes in brain structures associated with dementia.

Researchers are still working to discover what aspect of obesity might play a role in an individual's likelihood of developing Alzheimer's. A study out of Kaiser-Permanente in California followed 10,276 people, beginning from their midforties, for over thirty years. The researchers looked at such factors as age, gender, race, education, smoking, alcohol use, diabetes, hypertension, and heart disease. They found that medically obese people had a 75 percent increased risk for the development of dementia; whereas overweight people, with a BMI between 25 and 30, displayed only a 35 percent greater risk as compared with people who maintained normal body mass indexes.

But perhaps Kaiser's most intriguing finding was—more significant than BMI, which represents the total fat level in the body—it mattered *where* that fat was found. Those patients whose fat tended to settle at waist level showed a 72 percent increase in risk for dementia development later on. This risk factor is known as *central obesity* and can be measured by skin-fold thickness. (Ask your doctor about measuring this.) Even those individuals whose BMI did not qualify them as overweight or obese, but whose fat was distributed disproportionately in the midsection, displayed a greater likelihood of developing Alzheimer's, suggesting that there is a more nuanced relationship of body weight, fat distribution, and the onset of dementia than experts first thought.

Obesity and Vascular Risk Factors

Obesity is doubtless a complex risk factor. Studies have shown that being overweight consistently and significantly leads to a variety of health complications. The most serious of these are high blood pressure, elevated cholesterol, and diabetes. Since all of these conditions may be risks for Alzheimer's as well, scientists are trying to untangle the web of interrelationships among these risk factors to understand their underlying physiology. Investigators from the famous Framingham study examined 1,300 participants for up to thirteen years. High on their list of objectives was an effort to assess the interaction between diabetes and obesity. All subjects were given cognitive tests and physicals at the outset of the study, and were determined to be free from dementia, stroke, and clinically diagnosed cardiovascular disease. Researchers found that both BMI status (whether one is nonobese or obese) and the presence or absence of diabetes were intimately related to a variety of cognitive skills. For men, obesity alone was enough to impact cognitive performance: the longer someone had diabetes, the poorer he performed on the cognitive tests. Such gender-specific results for obesity but not for diabetes suggests that the underlying mechanisms linking each to cognition may be different in men and women. The adverse effect of obesity on cognitive function in men may be related to an interaction with diabetes.

What about the interaction of obesity, high blood pressure, and cognitive function? A recent study of ninety healthy middle-aged and older adults who did not have a history of stroke or dementia examined precisely this question. As in the larger Kaiser Permanente study, investigators looked for links between central obesity (assessed by waist measurements), systolic and diastolic blood pressure (see chapter 9), and cognitive function.

In general, individuals with both a greater waist circumference and higher blood pressure performed most poorly on cognitive tests. People with a combination of higher BMI and blood pressure also performed poorly, compared with those who had normal-range BMI and blood pressure. Taken together, these findings suggest that your waistline and your brain are not that far apart.

Indeed, in the long run, the bigger the waistline, the greater the toll on the brain

So why is obesity so problematic as a risk for Alzheimer's disease? Our best answers are coming out of the lab, in the form of animal studies. My colleague Dr. Richard Pratley, at the University of Vermont, has found that APP, the parent molecule of the toxic beta-amyloid protein that accumulates in the brain of Alzheimer's patients, is significantly overexpressed (meaning there is too much of it) in fat cells, especially those fat cells found specifically in the abdominal region. Finding APP in this part of the body is surprising in and of itself. We know that the more APP is expressed, the more inflammatory reactions we see in the body; and since inflammation is one of the prime offenders in brains of Alzheimer's patients, it follows that by accelerating the damage inflammation causes, obesity might be a risk factor for developing Alzheimer's disease.

There is growing evidence from the lab that calorie restriction is the most basic anti-aging strategy out there. Calorie restriction leads to a lower level of insulin in the body. One controlled clinical trial found that overweight people who cut their calories by 25 percent for six months lowered their fasting insulin levels and, conceivably, increased their longevity correspondingly.

Beyond its effects on fasting insulin levels and core body temperature, the low-calorie diet also changes some, but not all, of the metabolic factors that have been related to longevity or aging. Evan Hadley, director of the National Institute on Aging Geriatrics and Clinical Gerontology Program, said that the findings from the CALERIE project (Comprehensive Assessment of Long-term Effects of Reducing Intake of Energy), a two-year calorie restriction clinical trial, raises more questions for researchers about the effects on aging of low-calorie diets that are maintained for longer periods. So far, these data suggest that calorie restriction might swing the pendulum away from cognitive decline. Separately, data from animal studies also suggests that calorie restriction extends life. But, as yet, no research on calorie restriction can yet support the hypothesis that calorie restriction prevents Alzheimer's disease.

What Is the Impact of Body Weight
after Middle Age?

All these studies focused on obesity among fairly healthy and active middle-aged populations. Senior citizens also worry about their weight. I routinely ask my senior patients about their weight. Many complain that the weight does not come off as easily as it once did and want to have their stylish figures from earlier in life.

Ironically, I may be the only doctor in Phoenix who counsels his patients *not to* lose weight, but only in my geriatric patients. The reason for this is that losing weight in midlife is good; losing weight (especially involuntarily) in later life is *not* good. In fact, becoming underweight in later life appears to increase dementia risk. I have felt for a long time that unintentional or unplanned weight loss is generally a bad sign in the elderly, and recent studies support that notion. Elderly people who lose weight unintentionally are more likely to develop Alzheimer's than do those who maintain or gain weight. A ten-year study of Catholic clergy found that each unit decline in the body mass index was associated with a 35 percent increase in risk of Alzheimer's. Even before the onset of Alzheimer's, weight loss that occurs spontaneously without effort correlates with mild cognitive impairment in the elderly. One study published in 2006 shows that the effects of aging in those with and without Alzheimer's are associated with unplanned weight loss. This study finds that weight loss often accelerates just before Alzheimer's is diagnosed. Even before a diagnosis of Alzheimer's, investigators found that patients who had not planned to lose weight were losing weight twice as fast as others who did not have this disease. This suggests that spontaneous unintentional weight loss may be a preclinical indicator of Alzheimer's disease.

In the Honolulu-Asia Aging Study, a thirty-two-year study of nearly 1,900 Japanese American men, a high proportion of the participants who developed dementia lost up to 10 percent of their body weight in the two to four years before the onset of dementia. Researchers ruled out other illnesses and health conditions and concluded that late-life weight loss is closely linked with the onset of dementia.

Researchers from the Cardiovascular Health Cognition Study found that late-life obesity has a marginally protective effect against the development of dementia and that being underweight in late life appears to increase dementia risk. Being underweight in late life was associated with a 70 percent increased risk of dementia. Being underweight at age fifty, on the other hand, was not associated with the development of dementia. In contrast with the findings about those who were obese in middle age, researchers found that being obese in late life was associated with a 38 percent *decreased* risk of dementia. Researchers cautioned that the "obesity paradox"—the observation that excess weight may be protective for some diseases in the elderly—may, in part, be explained here by the possibility that physical signs of dementia in older patients, such as weight loss leading to being underweight, may occur before cognitive symptoms develop.

One hypothesis that may explain why this might occur is that inexplicable weight loss later in life represents a risk factor for Alzheimer's. But because significant weight loss is a common occurrence in diagnosed Alzheimer's patients, it is probable that the same factors that contribute to the development of Alzheimer's also contribute to weight loss. A third possibility is that the centers of the brain that are responsible for weight and satiety (feeling full from a meal or when we feel hungry) might be affected by Alzheimer's pathology even before the decline of cognitive functions is apparent with the onset of dementia.

Findings from both these studies should be embraced with caution; both the study of clergy and the Honolulu-Asia study used fairly homogeneous populations, so some of the conclusions may not be applicable to the general population at large. Also, just because an elderly person loses weight does not mean that he or she will automatically develop Alzheimer's disease. In fact, if I see an elderly patient who unintentionally or inexplicably begins to lose weight, I immediately suspect cancer or side effects from medications, not Alzheimer's. Besides these two culprits, there are many other reasons that a senior could lose weight. Depression, loss of the sense of smell (called *anosmia*), medications, and Parkinson's disease are among the most common possibilities. Many medications may cause loss of appetite and/or nausea as a side effect. Seniors also might lose weight if they live alone and do not have access to proper nutrition and meal choices. Still, physicians and family members should watch for weight loss as a possible cue before the onset of dementia. Weight loss might also be a indicator of other problems such as swallowing difficulties which might, in turn, warrant a more careful evaluation. Swallowing difficulties can also result in aspiration and resultant pneumonia.

A New Threat: The Metabolic Syndrome

The *metabolic syndrome*, also known as *syndrome X*, is a common condition in the United States and a significant risk factor for heart attacks and strokes. Now it appears to be a risk factor for Alzheimer's. The metabolic syndrome is characterized by resistance to insulin, high blood pressure, and elevated blood lipids/cholesterol.

Physicians now recognize a triad of diseases that include insulin resistance (type 2 diabetes), high cholesterol, and hypertension in the setting of obesity. This triad in the setting of obesity is called the metabolic syndrome. To have the metabolic syndrome, you need to have these three conditions, have a BMI greater than 30, and have a large waistline (40 inches or more for men, 35 inches or more for women).

The metabolic syndrome has now been linked to cognitive decline and Alzheimer's disease. In a five-year study published in the *Journal of the American Medical Association*, Dr. Kristine Yaffe and colleagues investigated the effect of the metabolic syndrome on cognitive decline in more than 2,600 individuals with an average age of seventy-four. Participants with the metabolic syndrome were 20 percent more likely to develop Alzheimer's than were people without the metabolic syndrome. In another study from Finland of nearly one thousand elderly, investigators found that people with the metabolic syndrome had an almost 300 percent increased risk for having Alzheimer's, compared to those without the metabolic syndrome. In yet another study of fifty patients with Alzheimer's and seventy-five matched controls, having the metabolic syndrome increased the risk three- to sevenfold for developing Alzheimer's. This makes it a potent risk factor and a great target for intervention.

Although we are still learning about the relationship of body weight, obesity, and Alzheimer's, managing your body weight and keeping it within a healthy range is key to cognitive health. Body weight is tied to many of the other health issues that I address in this book; and, as research progresses, the interrelatedness of body weight, obesity, and vascular and brain health grows only deeper. Reducing your weight to a normal range (a BMI of less than 25) is an important and achievable goal, as it significantly lowers your risk of diseases such as high cholesterol, diabetes, and, in many cases, Alzheimer's.

Final Thoughts and Recommendations

- Obesity is a risk factor for developing Alzheimer's disease. This risk can begin decades before symptoms occur.
- Obesity may double the risk of developing Alzheimer's.
- Obesity, when accompanied by high blood pressure and high cholesterol, increases the risk for Alzheimer's up to sixfold.
- Obesity, in the context of the metabolic syndrome, increases the risk for Alzheimer's even more.
- Obesity causes inflammatory changes in the body. It also may trigger the cascade of Alzheimer-type changes in the brain.
- Know your BMI. Your target is a BMI of less than or equal to 25 both for general health and for brain health. Ask your doctor for concrete ways to achieve this.
- Nondeliberate weight loss in the elderly is a signal that Alzheimer's or another serious medical condition may be developing.

7

Stroke, Cerebrovascular Disease, and Heart Disease

S troke is the third leading cause of death in the United States. Stroke is also the leading cause of physical and mental disability after the age of fifty and, as mentioned in chapter 1, it is also a common cause of dementia itself.

Stroke and Cerebrovascular Disease as a Contributor to Alzheimer's Disease

There are several types of stroke, including *thrombotic* (involving blockage of arteries that then deprives brain tissue of blood flow and oxygen), *embolic* (involving a clot that breaks off from the heart or the aorta and goes to the brain, causing brain tissue to die by blocking off critical blood flow), *hemorrhagic* (involving bleeding outside of blood vessels, leading directly to damage of brain tissue), and *lacunar* (small strokes usually deep in the brain, often related to high blood pressure). The most commonly recognized strokes are caused by blockages in arteries going to the brain. The largest of these is the carotid in the neck, but a blockage can involve other arteries both in the neck and inside the skull.

Not all narrowing of blood vessels going to the brain leads to stroke. Stroke occurs only when the blood vessels are actually blocked or burst. The term *cerebrovascular disease* refers to any thickening and narrowing of blood vessels in the brain that leads to decreased blood flow. With the decrease in blood flow there is an increase in the risk for dementia, cognitive decline, and even Alzheimer's.

In other words, could Alzheimer's disease be just a severe series of mini-strokes or the result of bad circulation? This was the common wisdom among members of the medical community at the turn of the nineteenth century. For many years, *atherosclerosis* (buildup of blockages in arteries) was held accountable for both senile dementia and Alzheimer's disease, although this theory was disputed by Dr. Alois Alzheimer himself in 1910. Medical textbooks from the first half of the twentieth century continued to regard *arteriosclerosis* (blockage and hardening of the arteries) as a general cause of aging, as exemplified between 1920 and 1947 in the medical textbook *The Principles and Practice of Medicine*, which stated, "Old age is largely a question of the blood vessels," and which also continued to regard cerebral arteriosclerosis as a major cause of senile dementia. This was considered an irrefutable fact until a series of brain autopsy studies performed in the middle of the twentieth century showed an inconstant relationship between cerebral atherosclerosis and Alzheimer's.

Clearly, strokes can cause dementia. The term *multiinfarct dementia* (currently known as *vascular dementia*) was proposed to describe dementia caused by damage sustained by blood vessels— "infarcts" (or strokes)—and was considered rare among dementias. Presently, vascular dementia is considered as the second or third leading cause of dementia in the United States and can occur separately from Alzheimer's, although there is considerable overlap. Strokes are also associated with other disabilities, such as weakness or numbness involving one side of the body.

What we really need to know is whether there is a link between cerebrovascular disease and Alzheimer's disease. Some recent evidence, including an impressive study conducted by some of my SHRI colleagues, suggests Alzheimer's research has come full circle. The work of Dr. Thomas Beach compared normal brains to Alzheimer's brains and found that *Circle of Willis atherosclerosis* (named for a group of blood vessels in the brain) was more severe in subjects with Alzheimer's than in control subjects. This is depicted in the photograph below.

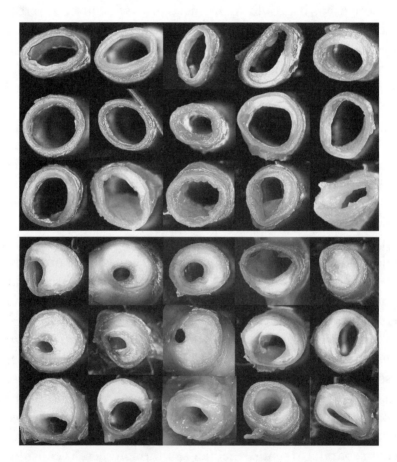

These are photographs of cross-sections of arteries with the brain. The top panel shows arteries from people without dementia. The bottom panel shows arteries from people with Alzheimer's disease. Clearly, there is a lot more narrowing of the blood vessels in people with Alzheimer's disease.

The top three rows are sections of blood vessels from people who died without Alzheimer's or any evidence of cognitive decline. The bottom three rows are sections of blood vessels from people who died with Alzheimer's. It is pretty easy to see that there was severe narrowing in the blood vessels. Those with severe narrowing were nearly *four times* as likely to have Alzheimer's as those with no narrowing. In other words, the worse the atherosclerosis in the brain, the more Alzheimer's disease changes accumulated there, too.

These findings prompted another of my colleagues, Dr. Alex Roher, to investigate whether this kind of narrowing could be detected while people were still living. To do this, he did a brain ultrasound (called *transcranial Doppler*) on approximately twenty-five individuals with Alzheimer's and twenty-five normal controls.

Dr. Roher found that narrowing of blood vessels in the brain was greater among the Alzheimer's-affected patients than in the normal-aged brains. The figure on page 102 depicts the difference: the higher the bars, the more the narrowing in the blood vessels. You can see that the people with Alzheimer's disease experienced more narrowing in their blood vessels.

In another attempt to determine whether Alzheimer's could be a series of mini-stroke events, researchers in Manchester, England, compared the occurrence of mini-clots traveling to the brain (*spontaneous cerebral emboli*) in patients with Alzheimer's disease and controls without dementia. Investigators measured the frequencies of spontaneous cerebral emboli with transcranial Doppler over the course of one hour in 170 patients with dementia (85 each with Alzheimer's disease or with vascular dementia) and 150 age- and sex-matched controls. What they found was striking. In the findings published in the *British Medical Journal*, spontaneous cerebral emboli were detected in 40 percent of the Alzheimer's patients and 37 percent of the vascular dementia patients, but only in 15 percent and 14 percent of their respective controls. These embolic events could not be attributed to carotid disease (meaning they could not be accounted for by narrowing in the carotid arteries, the big arteries in the neck), which was equally

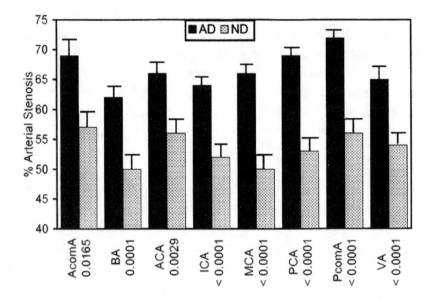

This is graphical data of transcranial Doppler ultrasounds performed on people with and without Alzheimer's disease. The higher the bars, the more the narrowing seen by ultrasound. Clearly the Alzheimer's patients (represented by black bars) have more narrowing (called stenosis) compared to unaffected individuals.

frequent in the dementia patients and their controls. The researchers concluded that such spontaneous cerebral emboli were significantly associated with both Alzheimer's and vascular dementia, opening a new avenue for both prevention and treatment of dementia.

In the Cardiovascular Health Study, which examined more than four thousand individuals for heart and stroke risk, those at a higher risk for stroke also demonstrated lower cognitive function at the beginning of the study and increased risk for cognitive decline during the course of the study.

Remember, decades ago, we used to call all dementia including Alzheimer's disease, "hardening of the arteries." Some recent evidence suggests that Alzheimer's has come full circle and that those who used the phrase "hardening of the arteries" may have been right all along but without fully understanding it. The take-home message is that the cerebrovascular disease from narrowing and blockage in blood vessels to the brain is a major contributor to vascular dementia and Alzheimer's disease. This should be managed aggressively. You can start by discussing aggressive stroke prevention with your doctor.

Certain Types of Heart Disease Contribute to Alzheimer's Risk

The term *heart disease* is very broad and encompasses many health conditions. Some of these include:

- *Atherosclerotic heart disease*—blockages and narrowing of the arteries of the heart that supply the heart with critical blood flow essential for its survival

- *Valvular heart disease*—narrowing and immobility of the valves in the heart

- *Arrhythmic heart disease*—irregular heart rhythm leading to inefficient heart pumping

- *Congestive heart failure*—an inability to pump as efficiently as necessary to prevent blood flow from backing up into the lungs

- *Cardiomyopathy*—weakening and immobility of the walls of the heart, which are made out of muscle

A "heart attack" is an event whereby the arteries supplying blood flow to the heart are blocked. This leads to loss of blood flow to the heart muscle that, if left untreated, can cause part or all of the heart muscle to die. Heart disease is the leading cause of death in the United States, but how is it related to Alzheimer's?

As I've mentioned in previous chapters, the more we find out about Alzheimer's pathology, the closer the connection we see between the heart and the brain. A number of studies have linked coronary heart disease with Alzheimer's, as well as with general cognitive decline. The link between heart disease and Alzheimer's was first observed about fifteen years ago when my colleague Dr. Larry Sparks was at the University of Kentucky. At the time, he moonlighted in the coroner's office and, during autopsies, he discovered that people with no cognitive symptoms of dementia whatsoever, who had died of a heart attack, nonetheless had Alzheimer-type changes developing in their brain. He posited that heart disease, cholesterol, and Alzheimer's disease were linked.

In one case-control study at the Mount Sinai School of Medicine Department of Psychiatry Brain Bank, investigators examined the hearts and brains of ninety-nine subjects who were devoid of cerebrovascular disease at death. Researchers found that coronary artery disease, and to a lesser degree atherosclerosis, had significant links to the density of neuritic plaques and neurofibrillary tangles in a subject's brain. This linkage was especially strong among those carriers of the APO-Eε4 allele. Other autopsy studies have corroborated that nondemented patients who died of critical coronary artery disease had more abundant senile plaques than did those who died of other causes. These results strengthen the current hypothesis that coronary artery disease contributes significantly to the extent of Alzheimer's-associated neuropathology in a patient's brain.

Furthermore, researchers at UCLA suggest that the interaction between Alzheimer's and heart disease is not coincidental. They found that people who have undergone angioplasty or a coronary artery bypass graft (CABG) had an increased risk of developing Alzheimer's over time. Comparatively speaking, individuals undergoing CABG had a 70 percent higher risk of developing Alzheimer's than did those who underwent an angioplasty/ stenting procedure without requiring a subsequent CABG.

The presence of the APO-Eε4 allele, as we have seen, spikes the risk of Alzheimer's in the presence of hypertension, high cholesterol, insulin resistance, or ischemic attacks. This further underscores the direct relationship between Alzheimer's and heart disease. Other possible common causes include incorrect cholesterol metabolism, diabetes, or high homocysteine levels. Each of these has been implicated in the processing of beta-amyloid and tau, the major components of neurofibrillary tangles, which I discussed in chapter 2. Distinguishing between the relative or independent contributions of any of these factors to Alzheimer's changes in the brain is difficult to research in humans. More animal studies are therefore needed to help us understand the precise mechanisms and factors in play.

It turns out that heart failure might increase the risk of developing Alzheimer's, too. A 1,300-person study at the Karolinska Institute, published in 2007 in the *Archives of Internal Medicine*, showed that individuals who experienced heart failure were at an increased risk of developing Alzheimer's disease.

What You Can Do

The same risks that lead to cardiovascular disease put one at a higher risk for developing Alzheimer's-related dementia. A landmark study by Dr. Rachel Whitmer et al., published in early 2006, revealed a strong link between midlife cardiovascular risk factors and a patient's chance of developing Alzheimer's disease later in life. Evaluating nearly nine thousand members of the Kaiser Permanente system in California, Dr. Whitmer's team looked at total cholesterol, diabetes, smoking, and hypertension. Having one of these cardiovascular risk factors at midlife (when patients were between the ages of forty and forty-four) bumped up the chance of getting Alzheimer's at follow-up between 20 and 40 percent, a probability that increased in a dose-dependent manner (the more numerous these risk factors, the greater the overall risk). People with all four risk factors were more than twice as likely to get Alzheimer's as were those who had none.

So what is the message here? Take care of your brain by taking care of your heart, and vice versa. As neurologists and cardiologists, it is our job, now more than ever, to make that connection when you come into our offices. But unfortunately, most neurologists and cardiologists don't see patients until disease or decline has set in. In the case of dementia, once symptoms have presented themselves, we know we are already too far down the path of Alzheimer's disease to reverse the damage.

This is why this book is so important to me. If we can raise awareness about the close links between the risk factors for cardiovascular and cognitive disease, we will give you the tools to lower your risk altogether, provided we can find you early enough. If we are successful, it means that in time you will be able to forgo trips to the neurologist and cardiologist altogether. As I said from the beginning, this is the goal: to work my way out of a job.

Final Thoughts and Recommendations

- Both cerebrovascular disease and stroke are leading causes of vascular dementia. They also put you at a higher risk of Alzheimer's.

- New research supports the old theory that Alzheimer's may be an extension of atherosclerotic events. It may be "hardening of the arteries" after all.

- Accumulating evidence points to cerebrovascular changes occurring in the brains of people with Alzheimer's.

- Coronary heart disease has also been linked with Alzheimer's, but the causal relationship is not fully understood, since Alzheimer's and heart disease share many of the same risk factors.

- Stroke and cerebrovascular disease are both modifiable risk factors for Alzheimer's; aggressive management of heart disease and stroke prevention will lower your risk of Alzheimer's.

8

Cognitive Killers

So far, I've talked a lot about risk factors, some of which are at least partly modifiable by lifestyle choices. In this chapter, we'll look at some events, disorders, and behaviors—"cognitive killers," as my colleague Donald Connor, PhD, calls them—that may affect your Alzheimer's risk.

Occupation and Toxic Exposure

For some of us, our jobs are on our minds from nine to five, but for many, our occupation is much more than that: a career, a source of income and of satisfaction and stress. But besides sick days and health care, how often do we think of our occupation as it relates to health?

The clearest way in which your occupation could affect your Alzheimer's risk is from toxic exposure. Exposure to toxic metals, gases, and chemicals can cause a wide spectrum of dementias and neurological conditions. Dementia resulting from toxic metals or gases requires either massive acute exposure or significant long-standing exposure to high levels of dust, fumes, or liquid through breathing it in, skin absorption, or ingestion. The workplace is the most likely setting for these exposures to occur. In general, dementia by means of toxic metal exposure has become rare, thanks to improved occupational safety regulations and the elimination of environmental hazards, but even where environmental regulations are in effect, companies often don't exercise due diligence on behalf of their labor force.

Acute poisoning can cause neurological symptoms that include acute confusion, dizziness, lack of coordination, and internal organ damage. In such situations, exposure requires immediate intervention. Permanent dementia may result from even a one-time poisoning, often as a secondary effect of brain injury from lack of oxygen. Occupations with the greatest potential for hazardous exposure include mining, smelting or foundry work, welding, plumbing, and construction. Any kind of extermination or fumigation, likewise agricultural work that involves handling pesticides, herbicides, or fungicides, can expose you to toxic loads that are dangerous for your body. If you work in manufacturing or are involved in craftsmanship that makes use of metals, glass, ceramics, paints, varnishes, or stains, you may be in danger if you don't take the proper precautions. Dentists and dental assistants who work with dental amalgams, which often make use of trace amounts of mercury, are also at risk. Car repair mechanics who handle automotive parts, chemical cleaning agents, or batteries need to be vigilant against lead exposure.

Metals associated with toxic exposure in these and other settings include lead, mercury, manganese, arsenic, copper, chromium, nickel, tin, iron, zinc, antimony, bismuth, barium, silver, gold, platinum, lithium, thallium, and aluminum. Some of the more common exposures will be discussed in this chapter.

Overexposure to carbon monoxide, carbon disulfide, organophosphate insecticides, and numerous industrial solvents (for example, toluene, hexacarbons, and hydrocarbons) can cause brain damage only after significant and repeated exposure. Poisoning can also result from intentional inhalation (sniffing or huffing) of vapors from volatile solvents for the purpose of getting high. Commonly abused solvents include toluene, halogenated hydrocarbons, benzene, and acetone; these may be found in common products such as glues, gasoline, spray paints, spray-can propellants, and cleaning fluids. As a recreational practice, inhalation of such substances can clearly cause brain injury, but it is not known if there is a link between this kind of activity and the development of Alzheimer's later in life.

Lead

Chronic lead poisoning is more of a concern in children who are exposed to environmental lead, usually in the form of paint chips or dust from old houses. In adults, sources of chronic lead exposure are less common but may include contamination from lead-glazed ceramics or lead paint, and occupational work with lead, including metal and ceramic work, construction, and plumbing. The risk of an actual dementia syndrome is present only when blood levels exceed 80 mg/dL. Treatment for lead poisoning involves identification and removal of the source of exposure and the use of chelating agents (medications to bind to the metals in the body) when acute confusion or other severe symptoms are present.

Mercury

Mercury is a particularly poisonous metal. It has numerous industrial uses. It is present in three forms: elemental mercury (also known as quicksilver), inorganic mercury salts (for example, mercuric chloride) and organic mercury compounds (for example, methylmercury). Exposure can occur by mouth, inhalation of vapors, or through the skin. Chronic exposure to mercury vapors in the past was associated with headache, fatigue, cognitive impairment, depression, and psychosis (the latter symptom illustrated by the character of the Mad Hatter in Lewis Carroll's *Alice's Adventures in Wonderland*. During the nineteenth century, hat makers used mercury vapors to make hats that would stand and not collapse; thus such workers would be exposed to large amounts of mercury on a daily basis). Since the turn of the twentieth century, mercury vapor exposure has rarely been associated with dementia and instead is seen in acute poisoning or in chronic over-exposure. Symptoms vary in degree, but can include neurological impairment (for example, fatigue, unsteadiness when walking, tingling sensations over the entire body, visual and hearing impairment, and tremor), and skin eruptions. If a large exposure is not treated immediately, kidney failure and death will occur.

The source of exposure to elemental and inorganic mercury generally comes from industrial fumes, thermometers, small button batteries, fluorescent lightbulbs, dental amalgams, and mercury-containing preservatives in cosmetics and antiseptics. Organic mercury compounds such as methylmercury, ethylmercury (thimerosal), and phenylmercury have also been used as pesticides, fungicides, and antibiotic preservatives in grain, house paints, and vaccines. Over time, many of these products have been banned or replaced in the United States. The presence of a mercury-based amalgam in dental fillings has not been shown to correlate with dementia or any other medical problems in dental patients. Those most vulnerable to exposure in this instance are dental professionals who are involved in the daily preparation of these amalgams. Methylmercury in the environment can come from both natural sources and industrial contamination. It can be fatal in sufficient doses.

Mercury has been shown to accumulate in the fatty tissues of certain varieties of fish, generally those fish like shark that are at the top of the food chain. Studies of women and children in the Faroe Islands, where diets are rich in fish and whale meat, have shown subtle correlations between mercury levels and neuropsychological impairment, suggesting that mercury exposure can occur even when the baby is in the womb or can be ingested through breast milk. Tragic outbreaks of mercury poisoning occurred in Minamata Bay in Japan in 1955, due to ingestion of contaminated fish exposed to industrial effluents. During a famine in Iraq in the 1970s, countless people were poisoned with mercury by contaminated grain. In both instances, individuals suffered severe neurological impairment, including unsteady gait, nerve damage, and visual disturbances, along with cognitive and behavioral disturbances.

Manganese

Manganese is a trace element and essential mineral involved in skin, nerve, and bone and cartilage formation. Along with zinc and copper, it plays a role in the production of antioxidant enzymes. Manganese toxicity is rare but may occur from overexposure to industrial or pharmaceutical sources, including manganese ore and dust from mining, and the manufacture of metal alloys, batteries, varnish, fungicides, and gasoline additives. Chronic manganese overexposure over several years has been seen mainly in miners. "Manganese madness" is characterized by psychosis and behavioral disturbances consistent with frontal lobe impairment (for example, mood swings and compulsive behaviors), followed by Parkinson-like features. Chelation therapy and the use of medications to treat Parkinson-like symptoms have not been effective.

Arsenic

Toxic exposure to arsenic and arsenic compounds is generally associated with the smelting industry where, during the manufacturing process, workers inhale fumes that contain the chemical. Factories that produce microelectronics are also a source of arsenic poisoning. Constant exposure to pesticides and fungicides, either through agricultural work or gardening, can also lead to a buildup of arsenic in the body. Finally, wood preservatives, coloring agents, and paints associated with home renovation or furniture restoration may contain arsenic. Acute arsenic poisoning can result in joint pain, muscle pain, gastrointestinal hemorrhage, kidney failure, and seizures. Chronic exposure can lead to mental confusion, headaches, skin and nail changes, tingling and numbness, physical weakness and fatigue, and an increased risk of cancer. Nerve damage in the extremities, the fingers and feet, can persist even after treatment.

Copper

Copper poisoning is rare and is generally seen only in the context of a medical condition called *Wilson's disease*. This condition involves a deficiency of the copper-transporting protein ceruloplasmin. This deficiency leads to copper deposits in tissues throughout the body, especially the liver, the brain, the kidneys, and the corneas. It typically begins with impaired liver function and progresses to include neurological impairment with unsteady gait, Parkinson-like symptoms, body tremors, lack of coordination, and slurring of speech in 40 percent of patients by their twenties or thirties. Without treatment, up to 25 percent of patients develop a dementia syndrome that includes behavioral, mood, and psychotic disturbances.

Carbon Monoxide

Toxic exposure to carbon monoxide is one of the most common poisonings in the United States and typically results from prolonged accidental exposure to fumes from vehicles or home heating devices that have insufficient or improper ventilation. Carbon monoxide poisoning can occur in or near a car left running in a closed garage or even in a room adjacent to the garage. A faulty furnace can silently poison people who live even several stories above the basement. The gas is particularly dangerous because it is odorless and colorless, making its detection almost impossible without electric sensors. Carbon monoxide binds tightly with red blood cells, leading to asphyxiation (starvation of oxygen) and death within hours. Individuals who survive CO poisoning usually make a full recovery, although a significant percentage may develop permanent effects including cognitive impairment as well as Parkinson-like features.

Removing the source of exposure is always the first stage of any treatment. Then cholinergic medications (see chapter 19) should also be prescribed immediately to minimize lasting neurological damage. If you suspect that you are regularly or acutely exposed to toxic chemicals, gases, or materials in your workplace or home, talk to your physician to see if a dementia work-up is in order. If you work in one of these environments, talk to your OSHA officer, get checked regularly by the occupational medicine physician on site, or go to the OSHA Web site (www.osha.gov/SLTC/index).

Medical Myth: Alzheimer's and Aluminum

About twenty-five years ago, reports hit the press about Alzheimer's being caused by aluminum. This news immediately resulted in a lot of stir, and people stopped using aluminum-based antiperspirants and cooking in aluminum pots and pans. The data from these reports were based on surveys of water supplies and on the fact that dialysis patients got dementia from aluminum-based dialysates, as well as on the identification of aluminum in the brains of Alzheimer's sufferers.

The research has not borne out aluminum as a risk for Alzheimer's. In fact, this theory was disproven by the research community over a decade ago. It turns out that there are many metal ions found in Alzheimer's brains, including zinc and copper, as well as aluminum. Furthermore, no link of risk has ever been established between using aluminum-based products (for example, cookware and antiperspirants) and development of Alzheimer's.

Still, to this day, I get a question about aluminum every time I give a lecture. This myth does not want to go away.

Sleep Apnea

Obstructive *sleep apnea* is a condition that occurs when the airway between the nose and the lungs (oropharynx) collapses or is obstructed many times during the sleep cycle. Basically, the brain is sensitive to the amount of oxygen in the blood. When sleep apnea occurs from airway blockage and collapse, the brain senses the declining oxygen level and sends signals forcing the person to wake.

People with severe sleep apnea can wake dozens or even hundreds of times per night, resulting in a constant state of daytime exhaustion and a constant desire to fall asleep. Sleep apnea has been linked with hypertension and with nighttime cardiac events. It is a frequent contributor to vascular disease and a known risk factor for stroke. Apnea has been implicated in sleep-deprivation-caused events such as motor vehicle accidents, and is also a risk factor for cognitive decline. While most frequently linked to vascular dementia, sleep apnea has been linked to overall cognitive deficits.

Overweight men with thick necks are the most at-risk population, but anyone can have sleep apnea, and other contributing factors may include a deviated septum, enlarged tonsils, or nasal obstructions. Trouble breathing during sleep, snoring, daytime napping, and morning headaches are all possible indicators of sleep apnea. Typically, a bed partner may hear loud snoring followed by periods of no breathing at all (as if the sleeper had died), followed by loud gasping and resumption of normal breathing. If you experience any combination of these, you should ask your doctor whether sleep apnea is a possible cause and if you are diagnosed with it, you need to pursue treatment.

Diagnosis involves undergoing a sleep evaluation called a *sleep study*. In medical parlance, it is called a *polysomnogram* (PSG). The typical PSG involves spending the night in a sleep lab, where technicians wire you from head to toe and monitor you while having a camera record your sleep. The PSG can detect how much oxygen you are getting and how many times a night you are waking.

Treatment for obstructive sleep apnea most frequently involves a continuous positive airway pressure device also known as a CPAP machine, which blows warm humidified air into your mouth and nose through a mask. To be honest, only about half of people tolerate this machine, but the half that do improve greatly. There are also surgical alternatives to the CPAP machine that involve reconstructing your airway.

Depression

Depression and depressive symptoms are common in people with Alzheimer's. Often, these symptoms have been observed soon before the emergence of memory problems that manifest in the early stages of the disease and may indeed represent the earliest symptoms of dementia. To study this association, the Multi-Institutional Research in Alzheimer's Genetic Epidemiology (MIRAGE) group, which I belong to, examined almost two thousand individuals with Alzheimer's and more than two thousand of their unaffected relatives. We found a significant link between developing depressive symptoms and developing Alzheimer's disease. Those diagnosed with Alzheimer's were more than twice as likely to have shown symptoms of depression in the year prior to diagnosis than were their nondemented relatives. But perhaps more fascinating, signs of depressions early in life—up to twenty-five years before a diagnosis of Alzheimer's—were a significant predictor of Alzheimer's. Drawing directly from the report, my colleagues concluded that depression is a risk factor for later development of Alzheimer's disease.

In a study of five hundred elderly individuals in Leiden, the Netherlands, Dutch researchers found that symptoms of depression accelerated in those who also had lower memory and attention scores. This was one of several studies that explored the link between patients who have a history of depression and those who later developed Alzheimer's.

These studies have concluded that depressives have at least a 70 percent greater risk for developing Alzheimer's. Although Alzheimer's may well cause social withdrawal or depressionlike symptoms, all these studies were based on observations of depression occurring *before* the preclinical phase of Alzheimer's.

In a recent cohort study, depression doubled the risk of progressing from mild cognitive impairment (MCI) to dementia. It remains unknown, however, whether depression is also a risk factor for developing MCI from normal cognition. The group at the Mayo Clinic in Rochester, Minnesota, tested the hypothesis that elderly individuals with depression are at increased risk of developing MCI by following 840 nondemented and depression-free participants for twelve years. Over that period, 17 percent developed depression, while 83 percent did not. Those in the depressive group were more than twice as likely to develop MCI as were those without depression, even after controlling for age, education, and sex. The association between depression and MCI was stronger in men than in women, and carriers of the APO-Eε4 gene were at a higher risk for developing MCI than were those who were not carriers. Interestingly, there was no relationship between the severity of depressive symptoms and the risk of MCI.

The Mayo group has proposed several possible mechanisms to explain how depression could be a risk for cognitive decline and MCI. First, they speculate that depression could cause MCI by affecting the brain's chemistry. Or, perhaps depression does not cause MCI but is related to it by a third confounding factor, which could be genetic, environmental, or both. The third proposed possibility is that individuals who experience some degree of cognitive decline may develop depression as a reaction to their awareness of the symptoms of cognitive impairment. A final hypothesis is that depression could lead to cognitive decline only in the presence of a genetic susceptibility or other risk factor, an idea supported by the link between the APO-Eε4 genotype and depression. The connection between MCI and depression may well be a combination of some or all of these proposed hypotheses.

Only recently have researchers begun to look for a possible connection between mood disorders and future cognitive decline. As a result, the population-based studies pertaining to the link between depression and dementia are few. But both the Religious Orders Study and the Baltimore Longitudinal Study of Aging observed that subjects with depression were more likely than were nondepressed individuals to become demented or to experience cognitive decline. In a review of the current literature, low-mood seemed predictive of cognitive decline in late life. It seems that the link between depression and dementia, while not fully elucidated, is strong and deserving of more research.

Remember, Alzheimer's and dementia pathology begins long before symptoms surface, and the results from the MIRAGE study seem to suggest that the link between mood disorders could be forged in the preclinical stage, as well. Depression, although it may put you at greater risk of developing Alzheimer's disease, is highly treatable. And psychosocial factors, such as emotional and social support networks and low stress levels, have been linked to greater cognitive and emotional health later in life. So if you or a loved one is experiencing symptoms of depression, seek counseling or treatment. In addition to improving quality of life and aspects of your health, treating mood disorders could help keep Alzheimer's or later cognitive decline at bay.

Don't Box!

As a child, I used to love to watch boxing matches. Boxing dates back to the time of ancient Greece, where it was one of the events in the first Olympic games. Boxers are the ultimate athletes. But since becoming a cognitive neurologist, I recoil in horror when I see a boxing match because now I know how utterly damaging head injuries are to the brain. Brain damage is as much an occupational hazard to boxers as black lung is to coal miners.

We've known for decades that boxing causes some brain damage; in fact, the term "punch-drunk" was used as far back as 1928. The brain is very sensitive to blows to the head. Such blows that occur with boxing can stretch nerve fibers and cells, disrupting normal cellular function. Another possible mechanism is that repeated blows to the head result in microscopic strokes (microhemorrhages). This eventually leads to scarring in the brain and the disruption of the brain chemistry itself. The bottom line is that boxing is all-around bad news.

We physicians have fancy medical terms for punch-drunk, including *chronic traumatic brain injury, boxer's encephalopathy*, and *dementia pugilistica*. But the more research that is done, the more incriminating the evidence against this cognitive killer. It turns out that fully 50 percent of all veteran professional fighters have this condition, including the famous prize fighters Joe Louis and Sugar Ray Robinson. Indeed, dementia will affect 15 percent of all boxers within an average of sixteen years after the start of their careers. Risk factors include long boxing careers with high numbers of bouts, older age at retirement, and sustaining multiple knockouts.

We are only just beginning to learn why this occurs. In a study published in 2006, investigators measured spinal fluid of amateur boxers shortly after a boxing match and compared it with that of a matched group of nonboxers. They found that spinal fluid markers for Alzheimer's disease were immediately detectable and significantly elevated in boxers. This supports strong evidence for the presence of brain injury occurring even at that cellular level long before a boxer exhibits symptoms of memory loss or dementia.

But it appears that the chronic traumatic brain injury seen with boxing tends to manifest symptoms more typical of Alzheimer's or dementia than of Parkinson's, and boxing severely damages areas of the brain responsible for motor, cognition, and behavior. Motor problems might include slurred speech and slow and uncoordinated movements; cognitive problems include poor concentration, memory loss, and slowed processing of information. Behavioral problems common among boxers include irritability, lack of insight, and paranoia.

Studies have shown that boxers who have the APO-Eε4 gene have much more severe brain damage than do boxers without this genetic risk. And one retrospective study found that Alzheimer's patients who had a head injury that occurred before age sixty-five developed clinical symptoms of Alzheimer's significantly earlier than did those who did not report head injury earlier in life.

I use boxing as a particularly colorful example, and surely it is one of the most extreme case studies of the link between head injury and dementia. But as you read this, be aware that all major head trauma, including concussions, can significantly alter a person's chance of developing later-life dementia. Some studies indicate that head injuries with loss of consciousness can double the risk of dementia later in life.

Repeated head injury is not unique to boxing. It is a risk for any sport that involves repeated cranial impact, such as ice hockey, soccer, and football. One study of soccer players revealed that frequent head contact used to field the soccer ball (called "heading the ball") is associated with cognitive decline. In fact, soccer players who headed the ball frequently did worse on cognitive testing than did soccer players who did not head the ball. Even CT scans can show subtle but distinct changes suggestive of repetitive injury.

Although no one can reduce his or her risk of head injury to zero—life itself can be a high-impact sport—take precaution, and be sure to always wear a helmet in sports or recreational activities in which you have the chance of experiencing intense or repeated cranial impact, such as bicycle riding, horseback riding, soccer, ice hockey, and football. I always wear a helmet when I ride my bicycle.

Don't Smoke!

You already know that smoking is bad for you. Add Alzheimer's to the list of illnesses that smoking might trigger.

The link between smoking and Alzheimer's disease has generated much interest and research. Initial studies suggested that smoking might protect against developing Alzheimer's. But not all studies have confirmed this. In a study of 258 Alzheimer's cases, with 535 controls, the Canadian Study of Health and Aging demonstrated that there is no protective effect from smoking. Likewise, the United Kingdom Medical Research Council performed a case-control study of 50 demented patients and 223 unmatched controls. They concluded that smoking increases the risk of Alzheimer's for mild smokers (defined as fewer than ten cigarettes/day) by 40 percent and for moderate to heavy smokers (defined as more than ten cigarettes/day) by 250 percent. A meta-analysis (an analysis of all studies combined) of several European population-based studies found that the risk of developing dementia and Alzheimer's increased in smokers.

Other recent studies suggest that smoking may be detrimental. In a population-based study of the elderly in the Netherlands, Dr. Ann Ott and colleagues from Rotterdam University found that the risk of dementia doubled in smokers as compared with never-smokers, and the risk of Alzheimer's was even greater. Dr. Suzanne L. Tyas and colleagues from the University of Kentucky in conjunction with the University of Hawaii found a dose-dependent effect of smoking on increased Alzheimer's risk in the Honolulu-Asia Aging Study (that is, the more cigarettes smoked, the greater the risk).

My colleagues and I undertook a study to examine how chronic smoking affected the clinical and pathological features of Alzheimer's. We found that those individuals who were smoking cigarettes at the time of the onset of their Alzheimer's tended to get the disease eight years earlier and tended to die of it eight years earlier, too. This effect was not driven by the presence of an APO-Eε4 allele, as we looked only at noncarriers of the allele. The amount smoked, measured in pack-years (the number of packs per day multiplied by the number of years smoked equals the number of pack-years) may adversely affect disease duration in a dose-dependent manner (again, the more cigarettes smoked, the sooner the subject died). If the smoking ceased prior to the onset of Alzheimer's symptoms, then the prior smoking history had no effect on onset, duration, phenotype, or outcome, and previous smokers were no different from nonsmokers in terms of their Alzheimer's. Our study did not support a hypothesis that smoking somehow protects the brain from Alzheimer's changes, but instead complements epidemiological studies suggesting that smoking may instead contribute to the development of Alzheimer's. In total, smoking does not protect against getting Alzheimer's and smokers appear to develop Alzheimer's at an earlier age.

What You Can Do

To reiterate one of the themes I've emphasized throughout the book, none of these cognitive killers is guaranteed to lead to your developing Alzheimer's. Nor is avoiding head injury or treating depression a foolproof plan for dementia prevention. But this chapter has helped sort out some warning signs and cognitive culprits that could bring on Alzheimer's later in life. How can you protect yourself? Keep yourself free of unnecessary exposure to toxic materials and wear a helmet while participating in sports or avoid sports if there's a good chance of cranial impact or head injury. Take care of yourself, including your mood and sleep patterns. And stay informed as we learn more about Alzheimer's so that you can build the best prevention plan possible.

Final Thoughts and Recommendations

- Avoid prolonged exposure to toxic substances and materials.
- If you suspect you or a loved one has sleep apnea, seek a diagnosis and treatment.
- Treat depression.
- Don't become a boxer!
- Avoid head injury by wearing a helmet for contact sports and bicycling.
- Don't smoke.

9

Blood Pressure and Hypertension

High blood pressure (called *hypertension* by medical profession-als) is perhaps the most common condition affecting adults. Up to 60 million Americans have hypertension, making it perhaps the most common condition in adulthood. It is commonly found with and a major contributor to other medical conditions such as heart attacks, strokes, and kidney disease. The good news is that high blood pressure is easily monitored and relatively easily treated. A wide array of blood pressure medication is available by prescription.

What Is High Blood Pressure and Why Should You Care?

High blood pressure occurs in our arteries. Think of arteries as flexible rubber garden hoses. When water runs through garden hoses, they expand their diameter to accommodate the water and contract when there is no water running through them. When blood is pumped out of the heart, arteries are filled with blood and expand. They contract when they are emptied of blood. When a person has high blood pressure, the arteries lose their elasticity and become stiff. As a result, the heart has to pump harder to overcome the inflexibility of the arteries, whose resistance impairs the blood flow to vital organs. Parts of the body farthest away from the heart—the extremities—get less blood.

The consequences of high blood pressure are enormous. Having to pump harder, the heart does the equivalent of a body-building workout 24/7, and becomes thicker as a consequence. As the heart thickens, the risk for heart attack goes up. Another consequence of untreated or undertreated high blood pressure is kidney failure. In fact, high blood pressure is one of the most common reasons for the need for dialysis. A third and very serious consequence of untreated or undertreated high blood pressure is stroke—hypertension is a leading risk factor there, as well.

Normal blood pressure is 90 to 120 mmHg *systolic* (the upper number, the force of blood pumped through the arteries away from the heart) and 50 to 80 *diastolic* (the lower number, the pressure within the relaxed heart as it refills with blood). Prehypertension is 120 to 140 systolic and 80 to 90 diastolic. Hypertension is defined as a systolic blood pressure above 140 and a diastolic blood pressure above 90.

What Is the Relationship between High Blood Pressure and Alzheimer's Disease?

Many large population-based studies have shown a relationship between high blood pressure and greater cognitive impairment. High blood pressure may affect the risk of dementia. The preponderance of data suggests that midlife hypertension leads to both more rapid cognitive decline and a greater chance of developing Alzheimer's disease. It has been well established that the rate of an individual's cognitive decline is directly associated with both elevated systolic and diastolic blood pressures, as well as with elevated blood cholesterol levels (discussed in chapters 4 and 13).

Remember, if you have a combination of high blood pressure, high cholesterol, smoking, and heart disease or stroke, the risk for developing Alzheimer's quadruples.

The impact of high blood pressure is broad and lifelong. In one Swedish study of people seventy-five years of age and older, followed for six years, severe uncontrolled high blood pressure led to an 84 percent increased risk of all dementia, and even moderate high blood pressure increased the risk of Alzheimer's in particular. In another fifteen-year longitudinal study, also in Sweden, researchers found that people with higher systolic and diastolic levels in midlife were more likely to develop dementia later on. A study published in 2006 suggested that your systolic blood pressure is predictive of future development of dementia. Dr. Lenore Launer, of the National Institutes of Aging in Bethesda, Maryland, and colleagues have noted that midlife systolic blood pressure, specifically elevated systolic blood pressure, predicts future decline in cognitive function and dementia. They looked at a study that followed seventy-one- to ninety-three-year-old Japanese American men in Honolulu for well over twenty years, When they looked at the 189 people who had developed Alzheimer's or vascular dementia in that period of time, they found that the higher the systolic blood pressure, the higher the risk for dementia. People in the highest third (blood pressures greater than 140/90) had a much higher risk for dementia than did the lowest third (normal, 120/80 or lower). It seemed to be particularly pronounced in people who had never been treated for blood pressure. This suggests that the process leading to dementia begins many years before someone is diagnosed. Dr. Launer said their findings showed that prevention and treatment of high blood pressure in middle age could prevent dementia later on, underscoring the need for management and aggressive treatment as soon as possible. Now is the time to begin prevention.

Interestingly, current Alzheimer's patients have lower blood pressure than do their nondemented counterparts, and Zhenchao Guo and colleagues at the Karolinska Institute in Stockholm found that blood pressure lowers as the severity of dementia increases. The reason for this, and the causal chain, is not yet clear.

Possible Mechanisms

One of the mechanisms by which elevated blood pressure might increase risk for Alzheimer's has to do with the angiotensin-converting enzyme (ACE). This enzyme is excreted by the kidneys and plays an important role in regulating blood pressure as well as metabolizing amyloid; blocking this enzyme lowers blood pressure. ACE is not only responsible for high blood pressure, but might be associated with damage of the inner lining of blood vessels. ACE mutations could also increase risk by promoting cardiovascular disease, another risk factor for Alzheimer's.

A study done at the University of Pittsburgh showed that cerebral blood flow was restricted in hypertensive patients, resulting in lower cognitive performance than experienced by peers with normal blood pressure. This finding suggests how high blood pressure may contribute to cognitive impairment or vascular dementia, and presents a mechanism by which regulating blood pressure might also improve cognitive performance and brain health.

Another avenue by which hypertension might contribute to or precipitate the onset of dementia is ischemic damage (meaning damage from chronic deprivation of oxygen and nutrients) in the brain. As I discussed in chapter 7, each year, more evidence surfaces that connects cerebrovascular and cardiovascular health to the brain and dementia development. We know that high blood pressure can cause or contribute to breakdown of the white matter (the connections within the brain) by starving these connections of their blood supply, microscopic burst blood vessels, and cerebrovascular damage in the brain—all pathological indications seen more frequently in the brains of dementia and Alzheimer's patients than in normal brains.

Oxidative stress, which accelerates the accumulation of beta-amyloid and neurofibrillary tangles, might also be at work. The truth is, the mechanism by which blood pressure is related to Alzheimer's is probably a combination of some or all of these events, making the therapeutic challenge for physicians even greater.

Treating Blood Pressure

Because much of the literature links lower midlife blood pressure with lower rates of Alzheimer's, researchers must now answer this question: Can lowering blood pressure alone reduce your risk of getting Alzheimer's? Or is a certain class of medications key in this protective relationship? Drugs that have been used for decades to lower high blood pressure are now being put through their paces to determine whether they might be able to stave off Alzheimer's, too.

The Kungsholmen Project (in Stockholm) found that blood pressure–lowering medication reduced the incidence of Alzheimer's in the elderly. But the Rotterdam study (in Holland) found that, while blood pressure medication reduced rates of vascular dementia, the same medications did not alter the chances of getting Alzheimer's later. The Cache County Study Group, headed up by my colleague and collaborator Dr. John Breitner of the University of Washington School of Medicine in Seattle, examined incidence rates of Alzheimer's to see whether Alzheimer's risk is altered among those taking different classes of hypertension agents. His team followed up with more than three thousand elderly people who had taken part in Utah's Cache County Study in thelate 1990s, nearly half of whom had been taking medication for high blood pressure at that time. The drugs used included: beta-blockers (for example, propranolol, metoprolol, atenolol, nadolol, and timolol), calcium channel blockers (for example, verapamil, diltiazem, amlodipine, nifedepine, and felodepine), and diuretics.

When these investigators parsed the data according to drug type, they found that only diuretics and beta-blockers decreased the odds of getting Alzheimer's. After correcting for age, education, sex, number of APO-Eε4 alleles, and other potential confounding factors, they found that beta-blockers reduced the risk of developing Alzheimer's by almost 50 percent, and that diuretics did so by nearly 40 percent. Delving a little deeper, they found that specific subtypes of drugs seemed to confer even stronger protection. Potassium-sparing diuretics, such as triamterene, amiloride, and spironolactone, were associated with a more than 70 percent decrease in Alzheimer's risk. The calcium channel blocker dihydropyridine reduced the risk by almost half. The findings suggest that not all blood pressure medication have the same protective effect, and that potassium-sparing diuretics, beta-blockers, and dihydropyridine may be standouts when it comes to protective properties.

Previous trials have found similar results, while others have found that use of any antihypertensive medication at baseline was associated with a 36 percent lower incidence of Alzheimer's. But the Systolic Hypertension in the Elderly Project (SHEP), the Medical Research Council trial, and the Study on Cognition and Prognosis in the Elderly (SCOPE) all found that beta-blockers, thiazide diuretics (which are not potassium-sparing), and angiotensin II–type I receptor blockers have no effect on cognition in the elderly.

A European study called the Systolic Hypertension in Europe project (SYST-EUR) looked at a particular type of blood pressure medication called nitrendipine, which is a calcium channel blocker (such as verapamil, nifedepine, diltiazem in the United States). The study showed that people who took the blood pressure medication for two years reduced their risk of developing dementia by 50 percent and, when the study was continued for two years further, the reduction of risk continued.

Using health data of the Japanese American men who participated in the Honolulu-Asia Aging Study, a team of investigators evaluated the risk of dementia and cognitive decline associated with the length of treatment of high blood pressure, grouping participants by how long they had been taking blood pressure–lowering medicine (the groups were: never-treated people with hypertension, those treated for less than five years, those treated between five and twelve years, and those treated for more than twelve years). They found that each additional year of treatment was equal to a 6 percent risk reduction in the incidence of dementia. At least in men, this suggests that the duration of antihypertensive treatment is associated with a reduced risk for dementia and cognitive decline. Whether such a duration-dependent protective effect exists in women being treated for high blood pressure remains to be seen.

What We Don't Know

We are still working out the mechanisms by which blood pressure–lowering medication might confer protection from dementia for individuals who take them in midlife. At this point, such a protective association is particularly foggy in diuretics, since they do not cross the blood-brain barrier into the brain like calcium channel blockers do. And it will be important, too, to confirm that beta-blockers and potassium-sparing diuretic blood pressure medications prevent the development of Alzheimer's in actual clinical trials. However, such studies are unlikely to be undertaken because they take a long time to perform and are expensive to conduct.

We also need to know whether reducing blood pressure through lifestyle changes is enough to reduce your chance of getting Alzheimer's, or whether certain antihypertensive drugs have supplemental benefits when it comes to protecting your cognitive function and health.

What You Can Do

For now, the take-home point is this: If you have high blood pressure—meaning a systolic level greater than 130 and a diastolic level greater than 90—and are not being treated for it currently, see your physician to discuss possible therapies. If prevention of Alzheimer's is on your to-do list, ask your doctor specifically about taking the medications commented on in this chapter, if they are at all medically appropriate. Ultimately, treating high blood pressure for Alzheimer's prevention is akin to treating high blood pressure for heart attack and stroke prevention. Research tells us that the care we take at midlife profoundly influences our chance to dodge Alzheimer's later on.

Final Thoughts and Recommendations

- High blood pressure is an independent risk for the development of Alzheimer's. The risk is even apparent in midlife, with consequences decades later.

- Studies have shown that rigorous treatment of high blood pressure reduces the risk for developing Alzheimer's.

- Keep your systolic blood pressure under 130 and your diastolic blood pressure under 90. This is good for your heart and your brain.

- Not all blood pressure medications seem to reduce Alzheimer's risk. Blood pressure medications that may include thiazide diuretics, beta-blockers, and certain types of calcium channel blockers (nitrendepine—available in Europe)

- Ask your physician whether these options are right for you.

10

Estrogen and Hormone Replacement Therapy

W hen it comes to the last decade of women's medicine, estrogen replacement therapy must surely be called the homecoming queen. Once thought to be a sex hormone only, estrogen has been shown to be a powerful actor in a wide array of human behavioral and biological processes.

But as a medication, estrogen's glowing reputation was recently sullied by a new and indicting spate of reports, most notably the Women's Health Initiative trials, which showed estrogen and hormone replacement therapy (HRT) to be a trickier business than believed at first sight, having harmful health effects that may outweigh any benefits it might confer.

This is certainly the case when it comes to Alzheimer's and dementia research. Initially a few series of case-control and epidemiological studies suggested that estrogen may have salutary effects on cognitive health in older women after menopause. This evidence has since been refuted by a bigger number of large-scale, well-designed studies that showed estrogen offered no cognitive protection and even increased risk for developing dementia and Alzheimer's disease.

In this chapter, we'll look at the research that's out there, examine a few hypotheses as to how hormones might affect dementia pathology, and explain why, for now, when it comes to estrogen replacement therapy, it seems best to sit on the sidelines.

Estrogen's Effects on the Brain and Alzheimer's Protection: Possible Mechanisms

For decades, estrogen was thought of only as a sex hormone that plays a fundamental role in regulating women's behavioral and physiological events. Estrogens are synthesized in a number of human cells and tissues, including the ovaries, the placenta, adipose tissue (fat), and the brain. Before menopause, the ovaries are the principal source of systemic estrogen in nonpregnant women. After menopause, the ovaries essentially shut down estrogen production, and other sites of estrogen biosynthesis become the major source of estrogen. These sites include adipose tissue, skin, bone, and the brain. The short-term consequences of estrogen loss are the symptoms that describe menopause: irregular periods, decreased fertility, hot flashes, vaginal discharges, mood changes, sleep disturbances, night sweats, and changes in appearance. The long-term health consequences of estrogen decline after menopause include bone loss that frequently results in osteoporosis, increased risk of cardiovascular disease, and cognitive impairment.

In the laboratory animal and the petri dish, estrogen is a wonder drug. It has been shown to enhance the effects of neurotransmitters (brain chemicals that cells use to communicate with one another), and promote healthy neuron development, growth, and maintenance. In the lab, estrogen has also been shown to have antioxidative powers and has also been shown to promote the degradation of amyloid precursor protein (remember from chapter 2—this is a good thing) by alpha-secretase (meaning away from the production of the toxic beta-amyloid protein that accumulates in Alzheimer's-affected brains). In addition, it actually enhances the growth of brain cells that produce protective acetylcholine, the brain chemical important for memory. Estrogen has been shown to be important in the maintenance of branches of brain cells called dendrites. It has also been shown to increase the level of growth factors that help promote healing of brain cells and which are important for the general health of those cells. Estrogen might even protect against excitotoxicity (overstimulation of cells that eventually causes them to die).

Because of all the positive benefits that estrogen has on the brain, it makes sense to consider this hormone as a possible treatment or preventative for Alzheimer's. But let me remind you, the studies just discussed were not conducted with human beings; when it comes to people, estrogen has a much spottier track record.

What We Know

The link between estrogen and Alzheimer's has been investigated ever since it was apparent that women are at greater risk for Alzheimer's than are men. Estrogen was first proposed as a treatment for Alzheimer's over a decade ago. For a while, researchers believed that estrogen and combination replacement therapy had the potential to reduce women's risk for dementia and Alzheimer's, a finding that would be of great public health significance.

But even in 1998, the medical community was far from unified on this matter. A meta-analysis that year looked retrospectively at the data from ten previous studies, examining the link between estrogen and a higher risk of dementia, a lower risk of dementia, and no association with dementia or Alzheimer's disease. In 2000, another rigorous and comprehensive meta-analysis of published studies noted a slight if inconsistent positive effect of estrogen on cognitive health. Two years later, yet another meta-analysis concluded that, given the problems in how the original studies were conducted and analyzed, the association between taking HRT and dementia risk was still uncertain. The epidemiological study in Cache County, Utah, found that estrogen distinctly lowers Alzheimer's incidence in women who took HRT; women who were on HRT for more than ten years were 2.5 times less likely to get Alzheimer's, compared with those who did not receive HRT. Tellingly, researchers found that any beneficial effect disappeared if the HRT was begun less than ten years before the onset of Alzheimer's, suggesting that any possible neuroprotective effect of estrogen likely occurs in the preclinical stage of Alzheimer's.

In the past few years, the pendulum has swung solidly away from belief in a protective effect of HRT, toward the opposite view: results of several studies undertaken as part of the Women's Health Initiative Memory Study (WHIMS) indicate that not only is HRT not associated with a lower risk of dementia, but its use may be associated with an increased risk of dementia. In a study of a combined regimen of HRT (estrogen and progestin) and its association with probable dementia, Dr. Sally Shumaker and colleagues found that those taking the hormone combination were about twice as likely to have probable dementia, compared with the placebo group. In a later WHIMS study, which looked at the use of estrogen only for women who previously had a hysterectomy, they found that those using HRT had a 49 percent higher incidence of probable dementia during follow-up, compared with the placebo group.

Both arms of this clinical trial were terminated—estrogen and progestin in July 2002, and estrogen alone in February 2004—because of more cardiovascular and stroke events and concern over increased health risks for study subjects, including breast cancer and heart disease.

In addition, several clinical trials have been undertaken to determine the effect of estrogen on the course of Alzheimer's. Several well-designed studies later, the findings demonstrate no significant benefit on cognition or progression in postmenopausal women with Alzheimer's. But a recent study by Mayo Clinic researchers, presented at a large neurological meeting, suggests that postmenopausal estrogen supplementation—the kind that most women have taken for such symptoms as hot flashes—may not prevent Alzheimer's disease. Researchers analyzed data collected from more than two hundred postmenopausal women with Alzheimer's and a similar number of nondemented postmenopausal women matched by age. Although the study did not show an increased risk for developing Alzheimer's in estrogen users, it did not show a protective effect, either.

What We Don't Know

With its health risks firmly established, estrogen therapy now presents new questions for researchers, ones of dosage and timing: Does when a woman begins estrogen therapy and how much she takes affect her health risks and benefits?

The newest emerging evidence suggests that the most protective time to take HRT is during menopause. Postponing it might make matters worse in terms of its impact on brain cell health. A study conducted in Australia assessing trends related to the timing and duration of HRT use on cognitive function looked at the hormone replacement history, lifestyle, and health records of four hundred women aged sixty and older. Standard tests of memory and depression were performed on all the participants. These tests took into consideration such factors as age, education, mood, body mass index, smoking, alcohol intake, and history of cerebrovascular disease. Investigators found that women with a uterus and ovaries intact who started HRT before age fifty-six, as well as those who underwent a hysterectomy and ovary removal within five years of starting HRT, performed better on general tests of cognitive function and on tests that assess the frontal lobe than did the women who began HRT later. The earlier administration of hormones caused the women to perform better on certain aspects of the cognitive battery. Still, researchers acknowledged that a much larger study, one looking at issues of timing and hormone therapy, was needed.

Another recent study by researchers at the University of California–San Francisco asked whether postmenopausal women on an ultra-low-dose transdermal estradiol (an estrogen patch) showed any cognitive or other quality-of-life benefit after two years. At follow-up, there was no statistically significant association between cognitive scores and those who were taking the estriadol versus those taking the placebo.

Another outstanding issue that remains to be addressed, apart from the question of timing, is which estrogen replacement therapy is best. Many kinds of estrogens are used currently for HRT. These include synthetic estrogen derivative, natural estrogens, and bio-equivalent estrogens. Synthetic estrogens are man-made. Examples of natural sources include conjugated estrogen (Premarin, Estratest) and estradiol (Activella, Climara, Estrace, Menostar, CombiPatch, Prefest, Vagifem, Vivelle, Alora, and generic brands). Examples of synthetic conjugated estrogen include Cenestin. The bio-equivalent estrogens are derived from plant sources. The biggest plant source is soy (for example, Menest). All the studies have principally looked at Premarin with or without progesterone. Premarin is a natural estrogen derived from equine sources (horses).

If a scientific study is well designed and carefully carried out, it will provide answers to some of the questions it began with, but it might not answer all and might just point the way to new avenues of research and study. In the case of estrogen therapy, one of these new questions is whether early menopause and estrogen replacement therapy might influence the disease process and Alzheimer's pathology itself. We know that women get Alzheimer's more often than men do and that not all of that disparity can be attributed to a longer lifespan. In the coming years, we may discover that estrogen is a piece in that part of the Alzheimer's puzzle.

What about Men?

As mentioned, Alzheimer's is more prevalent in women than in men but only by a slight majority. So what does estrogen have to do with male risk? It turns out that it is not that simple. First, men actually do have an estrogen supply that might be giving them protection. Testosterone is actually converted, at very low levels, to estrogen in men. Second, men may also undergo a form of menopause (termed *male menopause*), but this is very controversial. One of the characteristics of the male menopause is the loss of testosterone, which eventually translates into a loss of estrogen for men, too. Third, the biology of estrogen and the male brain as it pertains to Alzheimer's risk and prevention is not well understood.

What You Can Do

Heed the warning of this research and the Food and Drug Administration: if your health-care provider doesn't think it essential, *don't* take estrogen replacement therapy. If you do decide to take estrogen, do so for short durations and use the lowest dose possible. Any consumption of estrogens, hormones, synthetic hormones, or bioequivalent hormones should be done under the careful guidance of your health-care provider. At this time, taking estrogen should only be for the purposes of treating perimenopausal or postmenopausal symptoms (hot flashes, bleeding, and the like). Do not take estrogen replacement therapy or HRT with the specific expectation that you are preventing Alzheimer's. The data just don't support it right now.

Final Thoughts and Recommendations

- Women are at greater risk of developing Alzheimer's than are men.
- Although estrogen has amazing protective properties in the lab, those properties do not seem to consistently transfer to humans.
- Hormone replacement therapy comes with a certain degree of health risk, perhaps including an increased risk for dementia.
- Hormone replacement therapy is also not an effective treatment for Alzheimer's once symptoms are present.
- The current recommendation is to consider estrogen or other HRT only after consulting your doctor and only for treatment of peri- or postmenopausal symptoms, such as hot flashes. These drugs should not be taken with the specific expectation that they prevent Alzheimer's.

PART III

Real Recommendations

11

Eating Your Way out
of Alzheimer's

What you eat does not simply affect your waistline—it affects your brain, too. In fact, diet may rank among the top lifestyle factors that will determine your risk of getting Alzheimer's disease and may be a fairly easy thing to modify to reduce your risk. The connection between diet and dementia is a growing research avenue, and an already large body of scientific evidence from population-based and animal studies shows that when it comes to Alzheimer's, what we eat—or don't eat—matters. In addition to potentially reducing your risk of getting this disease, the dietary recommendations I set forth in this chapter may substantially reduce your risk of heart disease as well and are ultimately beneficial to your general health.

Reduce the Amount of Saturated
Fat in Your Diet

You've heard it before: diets high in saturated fat are bad for you. Saturated fats have been implicated in myriad health problems, including high cholesterol, obesity, heart disease, and type 2 diabetes. Now researchers have reason to believe that the presence of saturated fats in our diets might also affect memory function and possibly increase people's risk of developing Alzheimer's disease.

Much, but not all, of the evidence we have for this comes from animal studies. In these studies, mice and rats were fed diets of different fat levels and then given learning and memory tests; the ones fed a high proportion of saturated fat displayed worse learning and memory than those on the lower-fat diets.

In one study performed on rats, investigators examined whether the adverse effects were from saturated fat specifically, or from any fat at all. One group of rats was fed coconut oil, known for its high saturated fat content, for eight weeks. Another group was fed soybean oil, low in saturated fat and high in unsaturated fat, for the same amount of time. After eight weeks, the animals fed the coconut oil had higher triglycerides, higher total cholesterols, and higher low-density lipoproteins (LDLs, aka "bad" cholesterol; see chapter 13 for more details). The rats fed the diet high in soybean oil did much better on memory and learning tests than did the rats fed the diet high in saturated fat. In another study, scientists from the Medical University of South Carolina fed mice genetically engineered to develop Alzheimer's a diet high in saturated fat and cholesterol, with a control group of mice who did not receive the fatty diet. After two months, the mice were tested for memory-related tasks. Those that had been fed the diet of saturated fat were not able to remember the tasks, but the control group could perform them. When their brains of the mice were examined, the scientists found increased levels of the toxic beta-amyloid protein in the mice fed the high-saturated-fat diet. These data suggest a link between diets high in saturated fat and the development of Alzheimer's changes in the brain.

Obviously, rats and mice are not humans, so it would be unwise to draw definitive conclusions about human pathology from such studies. Human life is more complex, and conducting such experiments in people is not possible without raising a host of biomedical and bioethical questions. Thus, we can only infer from these studies that a human diet of high saturated fats will have some impact on our cognitive ability. To complicate the picture, the modern American diet is very high in both saturated fat and sugars. Genetic interaction, obesity, high blood sugar, and cholesterol levels are all bad guys on the cognitive health scene, too, so researchers have more work to do to determine whether the saturated fat intake alone or one of those resultant health conditions linked to high saturated fat intakes is at fault for the memory and learning problems in the rats.

Researchers found that people who were APO-Eε4 carriers (described in chapter 4) and who also had high intakes of saturated fat had an increased risk for the development of Alzheimer's disease, compared with APO-Eε4 carriers who had a lower intake of saturated fat. The intake of unsaturated fats, on the other hand, did not appear to influence the odds of developing Alzheimer's disease among ε4 carriers and noncarriers. But researchers in the Rotterdam population study found no association between high levels of saturated fat intake and an increased risk of dementia, complicating what seemed to be a clear link in the rat and mice studies.

These finds are promising for several reasons, and open further research paths to discern the complex relationship among high-fat diets, cholesterol, obesity, genes, and Alzheimer's risk. But for now, such studies offer us an intervention that is simple and clear: very modest dietary changes, such as replacing lard and partially hydrogenated fats with olive or other mono- or polyunsaturated oil, greatly reduces saturated fat intake and increases your HDLs (the "good" cholesterol), a proven good-health move as well as a probable aid in healthy cognitive function.

Get More Omega-3s

Omega-3 fatty acids, aka n-3 fatty acids, are a subclass of those polyunsaturated fats that the body uses for maintenance, structure, and function of many organs and tissues in the body. They are important to the development and maintenance of many central nervous system (brain and spinal cord) functions. Fatty acids compose about one-fifth of the dry weight of the human brain and, of those, 20 percent is the omega-3 *docohexaenoic acid*, what we call DHA (You will hear a lot about DHA in this chapter and in chapter 18). Much of this DHA is concentrated in the nerve synapses (the connections between brain cells), which are the tail-like part of a brain cell, making it a vital player in *neuronal signal transduction,* (the communications among brain cells). Furthermore, DHA has anti-inflammatory properties that may be the protective mechanism that inhibits or slows the development of Alzheimer's. In multiple controlled studies, mice fed dietary omega-3 fatty acids, including DHA, displayed marked superiority in learning and memory, compared with mice that weren't fed these substances.

DHA is obtained primarily through diet. Good sources include fatty fish (such as halibut, mackerel, salmon, trout, sardines, and tuna), eggs, and poultry. Fish contains two important fatty acids: DHA and *alpha linoleic acid* (ALA). Epidemiological studies of dietary intake of omega-3 fatty acids from fish consumption have shown that fish intake in at least one meal per week is associated with a 40 to 60 percent risk reduction of developing Alzheimer's. From these studies, we can definitively conclude that a high intake of omega-3 fatty acids is essential for both neural cognitive development and normal brain functioning. Fish that is high in DHA seems to have the most risk-reduction properties. DHA has also shown to be important in preserving memory performance, in studies done on aged animals. Another important omega-3 fatty acid is eicosapentaenic acid (EPA). Food sources of omega-3 fatty acids are shown in the table on page 143.

The Chicago Health and Aging Project (CHAP) was a wide, biracial community-based study of more than eight hundred Chicago residents over the age of sixty-five that relied on dietary surveys to assess omega-3 fatty acid levels in participants' diets. The questionnaire asked its subjects how frequently they ate from a list of 139 different foods, including seafood items such as tuna fish, fish sticks, fish cakes, fish sandwiches, fresh fish as a main dish, shrimp, lobster, and crab. Weekly consumption of fish was computed, and simple and complex memory tests were administered in follow-up over an average of four years.

Good Food Sources of Omega-3 Fatty Acids[a]

	EPA+ DHA	ALA		EPA+ DHA	ALA
Fish (3oz. cooked)			**Oils (1 Tbs.)**		
Anchovy	✔		Canola		✔
Halibut	✔		Cod liver	✔	
Herring, Atlantic	✔		Flaxseed/linseed		✔
Pacific	✔		Herring	✔	
Mackerel, Atlantic	✔		Menhaden	✔	
Pacific	✔		Salmon	✔	
Salmon, Atlantic[b]	✔		Sardine	✔	
Sardines	✔		Soybean		✔
Trout, Rainbow	✔		Walnut		✔
Tuna, Albacore	✔		Wheat germ		✔
Fresh Bluefin	✔				
			Seeds		
Organ Meats			Flaxseeds/linseeds	✔	
(3 oz. cooked)			(1 Tbs.)		
Brain, lamb	✔				
Brain, pork	✔				
Other Foods					
Caviar (1 oz.)[c]	✔				
Soybeans, cooked (½ cup)		✔			
Spinach, cooked (½ cup)		✔			
Tofu, regular (½ cup)		✔			
Walnuts (¼ cup)		✔			
Wheat germ (¼ cup)[c]		✔			

Source: Figures adapted from USDA, 2003.

[a]Foods that provide (per serving) 10 percent or more of the adequate intake (AI) for ALA or the acceptable macronutrient distribution range (AMDR) for EPA and DHA (10 percent of the AMDR for ALA). An AI is a recommended average daily intake level based on observed or experimentally determined estimates of nutrient intake by a group of apparently healthy people (thus, assumed to be adequate) when an RDA cannot be determined. An AMDR is defined as "a range of intakes for a particular energy source that is associated with reduced risk of chronic disease while providing adequate intake of essential nutrients."

[b]Farm-raised Atlantic salmon have nearly identical omega-3 fatty acid levels as wild Atlantic salmon and significantly more omega-3 fatty acids than wild Pacific salmon.

[c]Standard serving size not established.

Investigators found that a weekly fish intake was associated with a slower rate of cognitive decline (10 percent) compared with a diet of less than one fish meal per week and 12 percent slower among individuals who ate at least two or more fish meals per week. Fish intake was associated with a slower rate of cognitive decline in mixed models, even after investigators adjusted for age, sex, race, education, cognitive activity, physical activity, alcohol consumption, and total energy intake. However, fish-stick meals weren't found to have the same protective effect as those with fatty fish.

In the CHAP findings, the protective properties of fish consumption could not be accounted for by other protective dietary habits such as fruit and vegetable consumption, but might not be as strong after intakes of saturated, polyunsaturated, and trans fats are considered. Therefore, the role that fish consumption plays in

---

Eating Fish: What Counts for Brain Protection and What Doesn't

What counts:
- Tuna salad (as long as it contains little mayonnaise, since most brands are loaded with saturated fat).
- Sushi made with tuna, salmon, herring, mackerel, halibut, or trout.
- Halibut steaks.
- Grilled salmon and salmon burgers.
- Lox and other smoked salmon.
- Sardines.
- Recipes that include the fish types mentioned above.

What doesn't count:
- Most boxed fish sticks from the supermarket. They are made mostly from cod. Cod is low in DHA.
- Fish and chips (for the same reason).
- Most fried fish takeout/fast food (for the same reason).

slowing cognitive decline could not be conclusively determined. Further study is needed before we can definitively say that fat composition is, in fact, the relevant dietary factor in slowing cognitive decline. Still, we can say that regular consumers of omega-3 fatty acid fish did experience reduced cognitive decline and a slower loss of memory function.

There are, however, other large population-based studies that have supported the hypothesis that fish consumption has significant protective power in a variety of neurological functions. One study found that quantified fish consumption from a dietary survey discovered a marginally significant reduction in cognitive decline in men who ate one fish meal per week. So while we haven't nailed down the exact biochemical mechanism by which long-term fish intake equals better brain health, eating one or more fish meals per week seems to have some protective power against cognitive decline later on.

The evidence that omega-3 fatty acids have brain-protecting power is growing all the time. Patients already diagnosed with Alzheimer's have lower levels of DHA as well as lower levels of the omega-3 fatty acids. (I'll talk more about DHA in chapter 18.)

Alternative sources rich in omega-3 fatty acids, particularly alpha linoleic acid (ALA) include: spinach, flaxseed, and linseed. There are other sources of omega-3 fatty acids (particularly ALAs) that are not as rich but provide somewhat of a good source, and they include black currant oil, canola oil, mustard seed oil, soybean oil, walnut oil, and wheat germ. Still, when it comes to brain health, focus on eating a diet rich in DHA.

Consume a Diet Rich in Colorful Vegetables and Fruits

Vegetables and fruits that are dark in color are also a good bet for maintaining your cognitive health. As a part of its "Maintain your Brain" campaign, the Alzheimer's Association compiled a list of vegetables and fruits that have been shown to boost cognitive health. Among them are the following:

Brain Healthy Fruits and Vegetables

CRUCIFEROUS VEGETABLES	NONCRUCIFEROUS VEGETABLES	FRUITS
Arugula	Bell peppers	Blueberries
Broccoli	Corn	Blackberries
Brussels sprouts	Eggplant	Cherries
Bok choy	Onions	Red grapes
Cabbage	Spinach	Oranges
Cauliflower		Plums
Collard greens		Prunes
Kale		Raspberries
Turnips		Strawberries

The key to these fruits' and vegetables' cognitive power is that they are high in protective antioxidants, and that is what makes them desirable. It's easy to remember which kinds of produce to select: the more vivid their natural color, the more antioxidants they are likely to contain.

All of us hear the buzzword "antioxidant" all the time and may not know why that is really good for us. What is an antioxidant and why is it important to us?

Breaking Down the Anti- and the Oxidant

Antioxidants reduce *oxidative stress*. Oxidative stress is a medical term for damage to animal or plant cells, and thereby the organs and tissues composed of those cells. Oxidative stress is caused by chemical reactions in cells involving oxygen and by-products of the breakdown of oxygen. Some of these breakdown products inside cells include superoxide, singlet oxygen, and peroxynitrite, or hydrogen peroxide. The resulting effect of these by-products is that they interfere with normal functioning of cells. When there is an imbalance between pro-oxidants (that cause the oxygen by-products to form and damage cells) and antioxidants (that scavenge these oxygen by-products and prevent cell damage), when the pro-oxidants begin to overwhelm the antioxidants, then the cell begins to break down.

Oxidative stress is suspected (although not proven) to be a cause of neurodegenerative diseases, including Lou Gehrig's disease (aka ALS), Parkinson's disease, Alzheimer's disease, and Huntington's disease. Oxidative stress is thought to be a leading cause of cardiovascular disease. It is also thought to contribute to the aging process.

Oxidative stress within brain cells has been implicated in the neuronal breakdown associated with the onset of dementia and Alzheimer's. Growing evidence suggests that oxidative damage caused by the beta-amyloid peptide in the pathogenesis of Alzheimer's disease may be hydrogen peroxide mediated. Oxidative stress has been detected in brain, cerebrospinal fluid, blood, and/or urine of people with Alzheimer's.

Since there is evidence from multiple sources suggesting that oxidative damage plays an important role in the pathogenesis of Alzheimer's, it makes good sense to seek a steady, diet-based source of antioxidants. Several epidemiologic studies have found that a high dietary intake of antioxidant nutrients is linked to a reduced risk of Alzheimer's and slower cognitive decline. While studies of vitamin C and E supplements have so far shown negligible impact on participants' risk of developing Alzheimer's, data from the Chicago Health and Aging Project showed that dietary vitamin E was linked to lower rates of cognitive decline, especially among APO-Eε4 carriers. The Rotterdam study also suggests that long-term dietary intake of both vitamins C and E has an ameliorative effect on cognitive health. In that study, this was most significant among smokers, suggesting that the antioxidative powers of these nutrients help block the pathogenesis of dementia brought on by the presence of free radicals in the body.

As was the case with the omega-3 fatty acids/saturated fat studies, most of the evidence we have of a protective effect from antioxidant consumption comes from data gathered in animal research. These have shown that animals fed high-antioxidant diets demonstrate superior memory, reduced oxidative stress, and fewer etiological Alzheimer's changes than do their control counterparts.

We already know that the consumption of fruits and vegetables is an important component of a healthy lifestyle, delivering to the body vital nutrients such as beta-carotene, flavonoids, carotenoids, and vitamins C and E. These nutrients are front-line weapons in the war against stroke, coronary heart disease, and a variety of cancers. Researchers in the Chicago Health and Aging Project found that vegetable consumption was associated with a lower four-year risk of Alzheimer's disease. People who consumed three servings of vegetables per day had a statistically significant reduction in their risk of developing Alzheimer's than did those participants who consumed less than one serving per day. Consumption of all types of vegetables except legumes (beans, chickpeas, and lentils) was also associated with a far slower rate of cognitive decline.

In other words, your mother was right: eat your vegetables; they are good for you. The more of the right type of vegetables you eat, the less cognitive decline you'll have. Analyses of each specific fruit and vegetable separately revealed that a number of them were associated with less cognitive decline, including sweet potatoes, zucchini/summer squash, eggplant, broccoli, lettuce/tossed salad, celery, greens/kale/collards, and apples/applesauce. Those who ate the greatest amounts of leafy greens demonstrated the lowest risk of developing Alzheimer's. The CHAP investigators concluded that regular and significant consumption (2 to 4 daily servings) of leafy green, yellow, or cruciferous vegetables had a protective benefit on age-related cognitive change.

In a thirty-year, longitudinal, population-based study whose results were published recently in the *Annals of Neurology*, researchers found that women who ate the most cruciferous and leafy greens showed a slower rate of cognitive decline than did those who ate few or no veggies at all. Interestingly, in this pool of more than thirteen thousand women, the consumption of fruit did not seem to affect the rate of cognitive decline nor did it protect against the development of Alzheimer's disease. The difference between fruit and vegetable data might be explained by the amounts of individual antioxidant nutrients that are abundant in vegetables.

That said, blueberries have consistently demonstrated their robust protective antioxidant powers in both the lab and in epidemiological studies. Blueberries and other antioxidant-rich foods such as spinach and strawberries have staved off or slowed cognitive decline and Alzheimer's disease, even more so than purified antioxidants in supplement form.

Indeed, fruit and vegetable juices may play an important role in delaying the onset of Alzheimer's disease. As the most abundant dietary antioxidants, the many kinds of *polyphenols* (antioxidants exclusive to plants) found in fruit juices can better protect your nerve cells against hydrogen peroxide than do antioxidant vitamin supplements. In a population-based study of more than 1,800 Japanese Americans in King County, Washington, researchers tested whether consumption of fruit and vegetable juices, containing a high concentration of polyphenols, decreased the risk of incident probable Alzheimer's disease. The participants in this study were dementia-free when the study began and were followed for up to nine years. The researchers found that, after adjustment for potential confounders such as heart disease, there was a 76 percent reduction of risk for subjects who drank juices at least three times per week compared with those who drank them less than once per week. The difference tended to be more pronounced among those with an APO-Eε4 allele and those participants who were not physically active. The researchers concluded: "Fruit and vegetable juices may play an important role in delaying the onset of Alzheimer's disease, particularly among those who are at high risk for the disease." What we don't know presently is whether fresh fruit juices bear any advantage over frozen or packaged juices.

When it comes to choosing fruits for your Alzheimer's prevention plan, I recommend sticking with the proven antioxidant powerhouses of blueberries, strawberries, and pomegranate juice.

Drink Green Tea

One ingredient that seems to have particularly potent beneficial properties is a flavonoid called epigallocatechin-3-gallate (EGCG). Flavonoids are potent antioxidants, as they are free-radical scavengers. They trap the bad molecules and prevent the damage that can occur as a result of those molecules.

EGCG is found in large quantities in green tea. There is considerable evidence from animal experiments and epidemiological studies that regular consumption of green tea may have a healthful cognitive impact by unleashing EGCG's anti-Alzheimer's powers of neuroprotection, neurorescue, and amyloid precursor protein processing that may lead to cognitive enhancement.

Diet versus Supplements

Those studies that have tried to draw a causal relationship between certain nutrients and cognitive health have arrived at different conclusions when the nutrients in question have been ingested in the form of a dietary supplement rather than as an unprocessed food. Most of the current evidence tends to suggest that long-term dietary intake of protective antioxidants is needed to sustain benefit. It is more likely that any anti-Alzheimer's benefits will accrue over time. This means that long-term dietary modifications will have a greater impact on your brain health than will short-term doses of capsulated supplements. And in many cases, we still have to find out more about the biological interaction between nutrients before we can authoritatively single out their brain-protecting properties. Such subtle and still-mysterious interactions may in fact be responsible for much of the health benefits to be gained.

The bottom line? If it's a choice between a carrot and a beta-carotene capsule, go with the carrot.

EGCG seems to have protective properties that both reduce toxic beta-amyloid generation and increase the critical alpha-secretase activity in the brain, which is critical to preventing the overexpression of amyloid precursor protein (APP) in the brain, one of the main culprits in much of the neuron-level damage in Alzheimer's disease.

In a recent study, researchers from Japan examined more than one thousand elderly Japanese (aged seventy or older) to determine the effect of green tea consumption on cognitive function. These participants completed a self-administered questionnaire that included questions about the frequency of green tea consumption. The researchers evaluated cognitive function by using the Mini-Mental State Examination (a commonly used office screening memory test). They found that higher consumption of green tea was associated with a lower prevalence of cognitive impairment. When analyzed by the amount of tea consumed, participants who drank two cups of green tea a day had half as much cognitive impairment, compared with those who drank three cups a week. The protective effects of green tea were not found in black tea or coffee. The researchers concluded that a higher consumption of green tea was associated with a lower prevalence of cognitive impairment in humans.

Thinking about the Mediterranean Diet

The Mediterranean diet is modeled after the daily diet in those countries that ring the Mediterranean Sea, such as Greece, Italy, and Turkey. This diet has been shown to protect against a number of major health conditions and diseases, including obesity, cardio-vascular disease, hypertension, high cholesterol, and cancer. Rich in vegetables, fruits, whole grains, nuts, and fish, the diet avoids the red meat and dairy products that are the source of most satu-rated fats in the typical American diet. Olive oil and modest wine consumption are also critical ingredients. One of the principal dif-ferences between the Mediterranean diet and the typical modern American diet is this lower level of saturated fats and the higher levels of "good" fats such as those monounsaturated and polyun-saturated fatty acids found in fish, nuts, and olive oil.

Now it appears that the benefits of the Mediterranean diet may go beyond the heart and lower the risk of Alzheimer's disease, too. Investigators in New York City tracked more than 2,200 individuals without dementia for up to thirteen years, with an average tracking time of four years. They gathered medical and neurological histories, performed physical and neurological examinations, and conducted detailed dietary surveys and memory tests with each participant. The survey included a detailed accounting of the amount of fruits, vegetables, dairy, meat, legumes, cereals, fish, fats, and alcohol each person consumed. Based on the survey results, they then gave each participant a Mediterranean diet score ranging from 0 to 9. The people were reevaluated every eighteen months. Those who adhered to the Mediterranean diet had a lower risk, albeit modest (10 percent), of developing Alzheimer's. The higher the Mediterranean diet score, though, the lower the risk: the highest third of the participants scored had a 40 percent risk reduction, as compared with the lowest third. Beyond slowing the development of Alzheimer's, adherence to the Mediterranean diet seemed to provide a link to a slower rate of cognitive decline, even after researchers adjusted data for age, gender, ethnicity, education, caloric intake, BMI, and APO-E genotype.

A follow-up study a few years later of the same group of participants looked at their adherence to Mediterranean diet. The investigators found that higher adherence to the Mediterranean diet was associated with a 24 percent lower risk for Alzheimer's. The top third of subjects who continued to follow the Mediterranean diet had a 68 percent lower risk of developing Alzheimer's, as compared with the bottom third of the study's subjects. This impressive protective effect was still present even after factors such as diabetes, cholesterol, and high blood pressure were taken into account. The researchers concluded: "We note once more that higher adherence to the Mediterranean diet is associated with a reduced risk for AD [Alzheimer's disease]."

Perhaps the most interesting outcome of this study was the credence it gave to the whole-diet theory. That is to say, that the sum total of all items in the diet added up to the protective benefit.

When investigators teased out the dietary nutrients involved in each person's daily fare, none was shown to have a statistically significant effect on a person's risk of developing Alzheimer's or experiencing other cognitive decline. But the composite diet score (the sum of all the individual items consumed) described a significant risk reduction. This led the investigators to conclude that higher overall adherence to the Mediterranean diet is associated with a reduction of risk for developing Alzheimer's disease and lent support to their hypothesis that embracing and consuming all components of this diet confers extra health benefits that cannot be achieved by the intake of single nutrients alone or in the form of multivitamins.

This survey-based study is surely not the last word on whole-diet science as it relates to Alzheimer's disease. But the findings are promising, and the Mediterranean diet itself is an early favorite, as it has already been shown to have other salutary and protective health effects, including reducing levels of cholesterol and saturated fat in the body, and promoting vascular health. If you haven't already considered it for your waistline, you may want to consider going Greek (on the plate) for your brain.

Stocking the Fridge

Does feeding our stomachs feed our brains, too? Early answers seem to be yes, with many new questions and caveats arising from each new study. As a dementia doc who has long been concerned about my patients' diets, I am encouraged by my colleagues' growing interest in nutrition, which for a long time was considered a soft science. The more we learn, the more interconnected our diet seems to be with the health of our hearts as well as with the health of our brains.

On one hand, this has given us a new set of research challenges. We now need to figure out the mechanisms by which specific nutrients work their health benefits, at the cellular, genetic, and molecular levels. Although we have a long way to go, what successes we do have make our jobs as physicians much more rewarding. When I prescribe more omega-3 fatty acid–rich fish in a patient's diet, I can be confident that, along with possible Alzheimer's

---

A Day on a Brain-Healthy Diet

Breakfast: Fresh blueberries with a glass of pomegranate juice and green tea.

Lunch: Tuna salad sandwich (low-fat mayo) on nine-grain bread, served with a spinach salad (easy on the bacon) and green tea.

Dinner: Brain-healthy sangria (see chapter 12) as an aperitif. Start the meal with a bowl of curried lentils (more about curry in chapter 18). For the main course, try grilled salmon drizzled with olive oil served with fresh/steamed vegetables. For dessert, a bowl of fresh berries and grapes, served with green tea.

---

protection, my prescription is likely to lower his or her cholesterol, triglycerides, risk of diabetes, and atherosclerosis. Telling a patient to eat more leafy greens or drink green tea and pomegranate juice may well mean much more for his or her health beyond its regulating APP-processing in the brain.

Moreover, dietary recommendations also empower us to become participants in our own health care. Most of my patients would agree that learning a new tuna recipe or stocking their fridge with staples from the Mediterranean diet is much more satisfying than standing in line at the pharmacy, waiting to fill an expensive prescription.

Our ability to maintain our own bodies and minds is the promise of prevention.

Final Thoughts and Recommendations

- Reduce your intake of foods high in saturated fat and cholesterol.
- Eat fatty fish (salmon, mackerel, trout, halibut, sardines, and tuna) high in omega-3 fatty acids, particularly DHA, at

least three meals a week. Fish sticks and fast-food fish patties don't count.

- Consume three servings per day of the vegetables listed in the chapter.

- Although fruit has other health benefits, only certain ones have demonstrated protective cognitive effects. Stick to eating blueberries (as much as you can eat, and blueberry muffins do not count) and red grapes.

- Drink two or more cups of green tea daily.

- Adopt a Brain Healthy Diet (partially taken from the Alzheimer's Association Maintain Your Brain campaign, www.alz.org).

- Consider adopting the Mediterranean diet.

12

Red Wine and Other
Alcoholic Beverages

Wouldn't it be great if that glass of wine with dinner was actually good for you? Well, keep reading: it might just be.

Before I explore this possibility; first, a word of caution. Alcohol consumption, of course, is everywhere. In our society and many others around the world, alcohol is both glorified and stigmatized, a cornerstone of life celebrations but also the cause of death and grief. In the United States, alcohol is the great social unifier, embodied both in Cheers, the bar where everybody knows your name, and the great social disease, embodied by AA meetings, where millions meet each week and say their names as an admission that they cannot fight this substance alone. Millions more suffer in untreated anonymity. Alcohol is also the leading cause of all major motor vehicle accidents and doubtless fuels a great deal of the violence on the streets and in our homes.

Stigma or social vehicle aside, alcohol is ultimately a chemical. When alcohol is ingested, it is metabolized by the liver into another molecule called *aldehyde*. Alcohol and aldehyde are well-known toxins to the brain, the muscles, and the nerves. The risk drinking large amounts of alcohol poses to your brain has been well documented. Too much alcohol causes intoxication, which results in impairment of judgment and coordination. At very high quantities, it depletes the body's thiamine (vitamin B_1) supply, causing a condition known as *Wernicke's encephalopathy*, which is characterized by acute confusion, as well as visual, balance, and coordination problems. Left untreated, Wernicke's evolves into Korsakoff dementia, characterized by loss of executive function (ability to plan and complete tasks) and short-term memory loss with confabulation (making things up to fill in the gaps of memory). Excessive alcohol consumption has also been shown to cause structural damage in the brain, particularly in the cerebellum and a structure called the *mamillary bodies*, the part of the brain responsible for integrating sensory input with motor function. If that's not enough, alcohol is toxic to nerves and muscles and can cause chronic balance and gait problems and increases the risk of hemorrhagic stroke (stroke from bleeding in the brain) and seizures.

But more recently, brain researchers have become interested in whether there is a sweet spot of sorts—whether a moderate amount of alcohol consumption might actually have some of the same therapeutic or protective effects on the brain that it has been shown to have on cardiovascular health and risk of stroke. From a handful of large, population-based studies, the preliminary answer seems to be yes. Compared with those who regularly consume large quantities of alcohol and those who consume none, individuals who practice modest consumption of alcohol may reduce their risk of dementia and cognitive decline.

In the recently published Nurses Health Study, which followed the dietary, health, and cognitive patterns of twelve thousand nurses between the ages of seventy and eighty-one for more than two decades, participants who reported drinking up to 15 grams of alcohol per day (about one alcoholic beverage—see the sidebar on page 158) showed markedly better cognitive scores than those who reported not drinking at all. Women who consumed one drink per day had a 20 percent lower risk of cognitive decline than did those who did not drink alcohol regularly. In other studies, consumption higher than 15 grams per day has been linked to higher cognitive and memory scores, but not enough women in the nurses' study drank at that level for researchers to determine the presence of similar effect. Researchers determined that the type of alcohol consumed did not influence the effect on cognitive scores, nor did the presence of the APO-Eε4 genotype.

In a series of two-year follow-ups with participants in the Monongahela Valley Independent Elders Survey (MoVIES), researchers found that minimal to moderate drinkers displayed both better baseline cognitive scores and less decline on follow-up memory tests than did those who reported no regular alcohol consumption. This finding confirmed earlier studies that showed modest drinkers had and maintained better verbal fluency and memory scores with age than did nondrinkers.

Investigators in the Rotterdam study found that participants who reported modest alcohol consumption had lower risk for both vascular and nonvascular dementia, with those carriers of the APO-Eε4 allele demonstrating the highest protective association. But in a Finnish study, carriers who frequently consumed alcohol were noted to have a significantly higher likelihood of developing Alzheimer's disease than did carriers who never or rarely drank. This suggests that APO-Eε4 carriers seem to be vulnerable to such environmental effects as alcohol and diet. The findings of these two studies contradict each other. This disparity suggests that the

---

What's a Drink among Friends?

When it comes to alcohol consumption, defining terms is important. Most researchers in the scientific community have agreed to define one drink as 8 to 12 grams of alcohol.

Here's how common drinks stack up, by the glass:
- 4 oz. glass of table wine = 14 g of alcohol
- 12 oz. bottle of American beer = 11.5 g of alcohol
- 1.5 oz. of 80-proof liquor in a mixed drink = 18 g of alcohol

interaction between carrying APO-Eε4 and consuming alcohol is more complex than we first thought, and that although a modest amount of alcohol is otherwise beneficial, having the APO-Eε4 gene and alcohol consumption may not mix.

Staying ahead of the J-curve

What we are learning about alcohol consumption and cognitive health fits a common medical model, the *J-curve* (sometimes also called the U-curve.) The J-curve is based on the principle that consuming none of a certain substance actually confers a higher risk than consuming a minimum or moderate amount of it, and that as the consumption level of the substance rises above a normative level, risk again increases.

In the figure below, you can see that the lowest risk for cognitive impairment is at the bottom of the J, a point studies have shown to be between one and two drinks per day (approximately

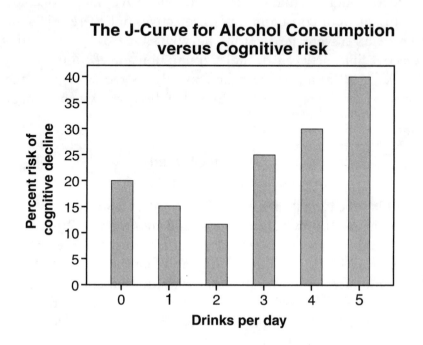

The J-Curve for Alcohol Consumption versus Cognitive risk

15 grams of alcohol), and that both nondrinking individuals and those who report drinking at above-moderate levels are at higher risk for cognitive problems and dementia. To be very clear, though, a modest amount of consumption may be beneficial, but anything more than that modest amount adversely affects the brain.

It is also interesting to note that the graph of alcohol consumption and overall death rate traces a very similar J-curve, with modest alcohol consumption representing the lowest mortality, then the chance of alcohol-related death increasing with number of drinks consumed at one time.

Is It Any Alcohol or Is It Red Wine?

At this point, it is hard to say whether any alcohol consumption is satisfactory or the benefit is specific to red wine. Most of the data comes from large surveys that simply quantify alcohol consumption and risk of cognitive decline or dementia, without breaking it down as to which alcoholic beverage maximizes the effect. Although the data is far from conclusive, most conclude that any alcohol consumption is protective, but there might be more of an advantage to drinking wine. One of the potential protective links between alcohol consumption and cognitive health is *resveratrol*, a substance found mainly in red wine and the grapes used to make it. Resveratrol has been shown to combat

---

"I don't drink that much . . . only a couple of drinks per day."

Quantification is important. In Sun City, I hear from my patients, "I only have a couple of drinks a day." When we talk further, it often turns out that the "couple of drinks" is not small in quantity and that they have several ounces of hard liquor per drink. In that context, a "couple of drinks" is far more than is beneficial to the brain. Thus the number of drinks is often not equivalent to the number of ounces of alcohol consumed.

the bone-marrow cancer myeloma and arrest the plaque development that occurs in Alzheimer's brains that was discussed in chapter 2.

Resveratrol actually prevented or reduced the growth of myeloma cells by causing the cell cancers to die through programmed cell death called *apoptosis*. When applied to Alzheimer's disease, a recent study in the *Journal of Biological Chemistry* suggests that resveratrol markedly lowers the levels of secreted amyloid peptide produced in different cells. While resveratrol did not stop the production of amyloid, it did promote the degradation of the amyloid. Resveratrol was shown to activate the enzyme proteosome to break down other proteins. This activation process is promising, since amyloid protection and plaque formation occurs years before Alzheimer's patients manifest symptoms. Long-term, preventive intake of resveratrol might enhance the clearance of the amyloid peptide before it ever takes root in the form of a plaque, and thus delay or even prevent the onset of Alzheimer's.

Red wine also contains *quercetin*, a nutrient found in garlic, onions, and apple skins. Quercetin has also been shown to have anticancer properties and in some studies has been linked to a decreased risk in cognitive decline.

The increased levels of HDL (high-density lipoprotein) in the bloodstream that moderate alcohol ingestion produces lowers cognitive risk by lowering confounding risk factors such as stroke and heart disease. This may be another mechanism at work. Or perhaps alcohol improves blood flow, which would explain its similar salutary effects on cardiovascular and cognitive health as well as stroke reduction.

Pomegranate Juice: An Alcohol Alternative

The health benefits of pomegranate juice are gaining attention. Not only is pomegranate juice high in resveratrol but it appears to have antioxidant polyphenols. Drinking pomegranate juice on a regular basis has been linked to lowering LDL cholesterol and reversing arterial hardening, a known cause of heart disease and heart attacks. It may even reduce the risk of heart attacks.

> **Brain-Healthy Sangria**
>
> Try a Brain-Healthy Sangria: Combine 4 ounces of red wine (cabernet sauvignon has the most resveratrol) with 4 ounces of 100% pomegranate juice; garnish with berries. (Do not consume more than one of these per day—and don't chase it with anything, either.)

One study from Loma Linda University suggested that administration of pomegranate juice to mice genetically engineered to develop Alzheimer's reduced the amount of toxic beta-amyloid protein found in the brains of these mice at autopsy. Thus it appears that pomegranate juice has multiple mechanisms for protecting the brain and body.

Proposing a Toast

Although researchers have yet to discover whether it is properties such as resveratrol or quercetin (found in red wine) or ethanol (found in distilled spirits) that is primarily responsible for the protective effect moderate alcohol consumption has on cognitive function, the dose seems to be the key factor. Remember the J-curve: risk for stroke, heart disease, and dementia is at its lowest between one and two alcoholic drinks per day. So raise a glass: it may raise your defenses against Alzheimer's disease, too.

Final Thoughts and Recommendations

- Drinking a modest amount of alcohol daily may have a protective effect on cognition and may somewhat decrease the risk of developing Alzheimer's. It has also been shown to reduce the risk of stroke and heart disease.
- More is not better. More than 2 ounces of alcohol per day can have harmful effects on the brain, including possible alcohol-related dementias or even stroke.

- Drinking red wine as opposed to other forms of alcohol may have broadly described health benefits, but its superiority in protecting against Alzheimer's is unproven.
- There are several possible mechanisms by which alcohol could lower cognitive risk, including ethanol or resveratrol, which has specific anti-Alzheimer's properties and is found in red wine and pomegranate juice.

13

Managing Your Cholesterol and Lipids

B y now, you are getting the idea that there is something you can do to lower your risk for Alzheimer's. In this chapter, we'll look at evidence that aggressive management of your cholesterol needs to be part of your health plan.

The link between high cholesterol levels and coronary heart disease has been well known for some time. So has the link between heart disease and vascular dementia (produced by strokes). Researchers are now trying to determine whether there is a connection between cholesterol levels and Alzheimer's, especially as it relates to the lipid-lowering drugs called *statins*. While this theory is promising, the literature to date is complex and by no means clear. Several large studies have shown statins to have a significant protective effect on cognitive health and risk for Alzheimer's; other population-based studies have shown no protective effect whatsoever; and, in a few studies, statin use was associated with greater risk of developing Alzheimer's symptoms.

I'll discuss these studies, including one conducted by myself and my colleagues at Sun Health Research Institute, and look into the biological mechanisms of cholesterol and *hyperlipidemia* (a medical term for high lipids in the blood) that may help explain why statins might be another tool in the Alzheimer's prevention kit we are assembling.

What We Know

The link between cholesterol and Alzheimer's risk is not accidental. There is an interaction that is supported by epidemiological evidence and scientific studies. This discovery has facilitated the possibility of using cholesterol-lowering medications to treat Alzheimer's.

Elevated Cholesterol May Be a Risk Factor for Alzheimer's

There is some evidence to suggest that high cholesterol may be associated with a higher risk of developing Alzheimer's. Recent studies have found that individuals with elevated cholesterol exhibit a greater propensity for Alzheimer's disease than do their counterparts with normal cholesterol levels. This apparent link has prompted researchers to investigate and establish a link between atherosclerotic heart disease (ASHD) and the risk for developing Alzheimer's. The resulting studies found that the lipid profiles of heart disease patients were, indeed, significant predictors of late-onset Alzheimer's and mild cognitive impairment.

Most of the data we have for the link between cholesterol and Alzheimer's falls into one of three categories. First, there are the epidemiological studies whereby investigators have chosen Alzheimer's or nondemented populations to look at the relationship among cholesterol, lipid levels, and statins. Second, as the medical community learns more about this disease, investigators can return to data already collected in wide, population-based studies to ask questions different from those posed by the initial researchers. In this data, it is possible to look for different connections between Alzheimer's, risk factors, and cholesterol than were perhaps reviewed at the time of their original studies. Finally, studies on laboratory animals can help tease out possible biological mechanisms between cholesterol and Alzheimer's pathology.

In the 1,300-person Finnish study I've discussed in earlier chapters, investigators returned to the data and found that higher total cholesterol levels at midlife were associated with a higher risk of Alzheimer's after the age of sixty-five, as assessed at the 1998 follow-up. This association was found to be independent of the presence of the APO-Eε4 allele. However, the risk of Alzheimer's for subjects with both the APO-Eε4 allele and high cholesterol was greater than it was for subjects with either the APO-Eε4 allele or high cholesterol alone. In summary, having both high cholesterol and a copy of the APO-Eε4 allele effectively doubles one's risk of developing Alzheimer's.

One group of researchers concluded that women with established coronary artery disease (meaning blockages in the heart vessels; known to cause heart attacks if severe enough) were more vulnerable to MCI when their total cholesterol and low-density lipoprotein (LDL) levels were higher. When, in these same patients, total cholesterol and LDL levels were lowered over a period of four years, researchers saw that their risk of cognitive decline was virtually cut in half. There was also an improvement in overall cognitive function, regardless of an individual's APO-Eε4 carrier status.

Some studies have implicated low levels of HDL, the good kind of cholesterol, as the central agent in Alzheimer's development. When HDL serum levels in Alzheimer's patients were compared with non-Alzheimer's patients, it was found that the severity of Alzheimer's correlated closely to the lower levels of HDL. The lower the levels of HDL, the more severe the Alzheimer's.

Indeed, evidence suggests that HDL may have a protective effect on cognition. In a recent study of almost 140 nonagenerians (people in their nineties) and centenarians (people in their hundreds), researchers found a statistically significant correlation between HDL levels and scores on the Mini Mental State Examination (MMSE), indicating that the higher an individual's HDL level was, the better was his or her performance on simple bedside memory tests.

Possible Mechanisms

Although big question marks are still attached to the link between high cholesterol and Alzheimer's, there is widespread support in the medical community for a proposed model that explains how *hypercholesterolemia* (high cholesterol) might induce Alzheimer's pathology. At the cellular level, cholesterol triggers excess production and secretion of the toxic beta-amyloid protein. As you already know, this protein accumulation is a central biochemical factor in Alzheimer's pathology.

Laboratory studies in mice bear out this chain of events. Several animal studies have demonstrated that increasing cholesterol in the diet resulted in acceleration of beta-amyloid deposition, while reducing cholesterol (either by change in diet or medication) reversed that deposition. Another theory is that accumulation of cholesterol accelerates oxidation (a toxic biochemical reaction), which, in turn, precipitates the vascular damage that has been well established as a contributor to the onset of Alzheimer's.

What We Don't Know

Part of the mystery regarding cholesterol's relationship to Alzheimer's is whether levels of "bad" cholesterol in the body have a distinct effect on Alzheimer's pathology, such as beta-amyloid accumulation, or whether the relationship between higher midlife LDL and total cholesterol levels and the onset of Alzheimer's is purely a connecting line between cholesterol's cumulative vascular effects and their proven effect on brain function.

Statins: Do They Do Double-Duty?

Although the studies that show this are recent and not unanimous, statins, one type of *lipid-lowering agent* (LLA) prescribed to lower cholesterol may also lower a person's risk of developing Alzheimer's. The first study to suggest this was published in 2000. By examining a cross-section of patients' medical records, researchers found a significant decrease in Alzheimer's incidence among those on HMG-CoA reductase inhibitors (statins).

Q&A: Cholesterol-Lowering Medications

Are all statins lipid-lowering agents? Yes.

Are all cholesterol-lowering medications statins? No.

What is a statin? Production of cholesterol can be inhibited by medications that inhibit the enzyme involved in the production of cholesterol (3-hydroxy-3-methylglutaryl-coenzyme A, or HMG-CoA reductase inhibitors). These are known as statins.

What does a statin do? Since statins are medications that block the key step for the production of cholesterol, they are powerful reducers of blood total cholesterol and the bad cholesterol (LDL).

Which medications are statins? Statins include atorvastatin (Lipitor), pravastain (Pravachol), rosuvastatin (Crestor), lovastatin (Mevacor), simvastatin (Zocor), and fluvastatin (Lescol). Sometimes statins are combined with other medications. Examples of this include simvastatin (Zocor) combined with a drug intended to block absorption of cholesterol, called ezetimibe (Zetia). This combination is branded under the name Vytorin. Another example is the combination of the blood pressure medication amlodipine with atorvastatin (Lipitor). This combination is branded under the name Caduet.

Does taking statins require monitoring? Yes. Statins can affect the liver and the muscles, although damage is infrequent. Because of this, your doctor should monitor liver activity with a blood test called *liver function test* (LFT) and watch for muscle breakdown with a blood test that measures *creatine phosphokinase* (CPK). When the LFTs or CPK go up significantly, your doctor should consider switching medications or stopping the statins.

What are statins used for? Statins are indicated as treatments for reduction of blood cholesterol levels in people with elevated blood cholesterol. Taking these medications has been shown to lower the risk for heart disease and stroke.

What are other cholesterol-lowering agents? These include fenofibrate (Antara, Lofibra, Tricor, and Triglide), nicotinic acid agents (Advicor and Niaspan), gemfibrozil (Lopid), cholestryramine (Questran), and ezetimibe (Zetia).

Do other types of cholesterol-lowering medications protect against Alzheimer's? We don't know yet.

Other epidemiological studies have borne out this finding. In one assessment of a national health registry in England, investigators looked at individuals who were at least fifty years old and met one of three conditions:

1. They had been prescribed at least one statin or other lipid-lowering agent.

2. They had untreated elevations of cholesterol levels.

3. They had neither elevated cholesterol nor a prescription for a lipid-lowering agent.

Analysis of this data showed that patients who were prescribed statins had a 71 percent lower risk of developing dementia or Alzheimer's.

Researchers in Canada reviewed the data from the Canadian Study of Health and Aging to see if there was an association between dementia and lipid-lowering agents. The original study examined more than 1,300 individuals for more than five years, during which almost 500 had converted to Alzheimer's or dementia from normal aging. The rest of them showed no signs of dementia at the outset and at the follow-up. They found that statin use was associated with a lower risk of dementia and Alzheimer's for individuals less than eighty years of age, but that statins' protective effect seemed to disappear after that.

Drawing on the data from the Cardiovascular Health Study (described briefly in chapter 7), a review of patient charts showed that at the initial office visit, patients on statins were less likely to have dementia or Alzheimer's disease. At follow-up—an average of ten to eleven months after the initial visit—patients in the statin group improved on simple memory tests, whereas the scores for patients not taking statins got worse. Twenty-five percent of the sample was included in this follow-up. This association between statin use and increased scores on these simple bedside memory tests is important because it points to the potential of statins to delay or even arrest cognitive decline.

The preponderance of epidemiological data suggests that statin treatment may also reduce the risk of developing Alzheimer's disease later in life. Since the initial epidemiologic investigation assessing the effect of statin use on later risk of developing Alzheimer's, there have been ten additional studies; all but two reported some benefit as a result of cholesterol-lowering therapy. Some of the conflicting results come from another report by Cardiovascular Health Study, which indicated that there was no significant reduction in the risk of Alzheimer's with statin use, but the investigators allowed for the possibility that some benefit could be provided with longer-term statin therapy.

My colleagues Drs. Farrer and Green of Boston University, who led the MIRAGE study group, have looked at statin use as it pertains to Alzheimer's risk, as well. This group studied nearly 900 people with Alzheimer's and almost 1,500 of their siblings who showed no signs of dementia. They found that the people who took statins reduced the risk of developing Alzheimer's by about 40 percent. Taking other cholesterol-lowering medications (nonstatins) was not associated with a lowered risk, regardless of the presence of APO-E, heart disease, diabetes, smoking, high blood pressure, or stroke. These data suggest that statins have some unique property that comes into play with regard to cognitive protection.

Overall, the evidence, with limited exceptions, suggests that statin therapy provides some degree of benefit, both toward reducing the risk of Alzheimer's in later life and in treating individuals who already have it.

How Statins Work

Cholesterol is known to be involved in the deposition of beta-amyloid protein in the brain. Some researchers have proposed that cholesterol interacts with the initial amyloid cascade. Drug studies are currently under way, looking at ways of influencing cholesterol metabolism. For example, simvastatin (Zocor) has been shown to reduce the cerebrospinal fluid and brain tissue levels of beta-amyloid protein.

When it comes to Alzheimer's disease, there are several potential mechanisms where statins might confer their benefits. They might work by simply reducing cholesterol, which we know promotes deposition of beta-amyloid protein by shifting APP (the parent molecule of amyloid) metabolism from alpha (leading to benign by-products) to beta (leading to toxic by-products) cleavage. Alternatively, statins could work by reducing inflammation. We have already discussed the fact that inflammation is an equal source of brain cell damage in Alzheimer's patients. The established antioxidative and anti-inflammatory power of statins in heart disease may have similar salutary influence on neurological inflammation in the Alzheimer's cascade, perhaps by reducing activation of scavenger cells called *microglia* that are activated to clear out the debris of the dead cells ravaged by Alzheimer's. Other mechanisms are likely, as well.

The Next Step

Our group at Sun Health Research Institute, led by my colleague Dr. Larry Sparks, performed the first randomized, double-blind, placebo-controlled, clinical trial to investigate the effects of atorvastatin (Lipitor) in the treatment of Alzheimer's. Essentially, this means that participants received Lipitor or a placebo, and neither the doctors nor the participants knew who received which. All participants had a diagnosis of mild to moderate Alzheimer's and were allowed to continue taking donepezil (Aricept), rivastigmine (Exelon), or galantamine (Reminyl/Razadyne) throughout the trial. The primary measure of the outcome was a forty-five-minute memory test as required by the FDA in Alzheimer's clinical trials

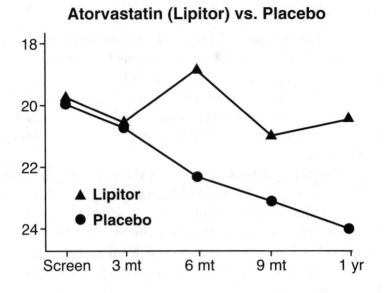

Differences in rate of change on cognitive tests between
Alzheimer's subjects taking Lipitor and those taking a placebo.

(Alzheimer's Disease Assessment Scale-Cognitive Subscale, aka
ADAS-cog).

We found that cognitive function in Alzheimer's patients stabilized. As early as six months into the study, we observed that the placebo group (depicted in the figure above by the black circles) had shown a steady decline (which was expected), where the Lipitor-treated population (depicted by the black triangles) showed no improvement—but no decline, either. This finding was significant in that it showed that the disease could actually be slowed down. As seen in the figure above, this held true at the twelve-month follow-up.

What We Don't Know

If taking statins indeed does protect against Alzheimer's, then the questions are: Which statins? When it comes to Alzheimer's, do all statins work the same way? And if they do confer cognitive protection, do all statins confer the same kind of protection?

These questions are all matters of great debate in the research community in the United States and abroad. One open label (meaning the patient and the investigator knew what they were taking) study done in Europe showed that Alzheimer's patients taking simvastatin (Zocor) showed slower cognitive decline after just six months of treatment. Except for simvastatin and atorvastatin, no other statins have been studied in this matter.

Another question we must try to answer is: Is lowering cholesterol levels or some other secondary effect of statins the key link between this drug class and Alzheimer's disease? Data from the MIRAGE study suggest that the protective effect was from statins and not from other cholesterol-lowering medications, strengthening the possibility that statins' anti-inflammatory properties might be the Alzheimer's-slowing link. An autopsy study of Alzheimer's brains demonstrated that chronic statin users had less activation of cells associated with an inflammatory response (microglia) compared to those patients who did not take statins.

We also don't know whether lowering your risk of cholesterol by other means, such as rigorous diet and exercise, also lowers your risk for Alzheimer's, and whether such a risk reduction is equal to taking a statin.

As researchers, these are some of the questions posed by recent population-based studies. We must continue to look for real answers through rigorous clinical trials, such as the one we completed using Lipitor as a treatment for Alzheimer's. We know that statins appear to stabilize the cognitive changes associated with this disease, but we still need to perform a good deal more clinical research to more fully determine whether taking statins actually prevents or delays the onset of Alzheimer's.

What You Can Do

Even though the research on maintaining your brain by lowering cholesterol levels by statins and dietary means is not unanimous, it is certainly promising.

The incentive to get your cholesterol levels (as discussed in chapter 4) monitored regularly and seek therapy for high LDL or total cholesterol levels is already there. This has been a critical part of heart health for decades now. Whether or not future research bears out an independent connection among cholesterol, statins, and Alzheimer's, the link between the health of our brains and our hearts is closer than we ever thought. As a neurologist, I wholeheartedly advocate checking your cholesterol levels and seeking lipid-lowering therapy, particularly with a statin. Some doctors even recommend that those patients with a family history of heart disease take statins as a prophylactic, even if cholesterol levels are under control. As with all prescription medications, this decision should be between you and your physician. Consider that statins may benefit your brain, too.

Final Thoughts and Recommendations

- Maintain your cholesterol as if you were treating it for heart disease.
- Your target total cholesterol should be less than 200 mg/dl.
- Your target HDL ("good" cholesterol) should be greater than 50 mg/dl.
- Your target LDL ("bad" cholesterol) should be less than 130 mg/dl (ideally, less than 100 mg/dl).
- Your target triglycerides should be less than 150 mg/dl.
- Taking a statin appears to reduce your risk for the development of Alzheimer's, possibly as much as 70 percent. This property is not apparent for all medications that lower cholesterol.
- The above targets and the therapies to help you achieve them should be discussed with your doctor.

14

Exercising Your Way toward Prevention

U se it or lose it"—we've all heard that phrase before. And now it seems that same sentiment applies to Alzheimer's prevention: emerging evidence suggests that vigorous and sustained physical activity is indeed good for the brain. It also applies to mental activity, too, and we will discuss that in the next chapter. Regular exercise and workouts may not simply benefit your muscles, bones, heart, stamina, waistline, and mood (isn't that enough already?), but there is mounting evidence that it could amp up your brain's power to fight Alzheimer's and dementia.

Another Reason to Renew Your Gym Membership

Physical exercise is essential to maintaining good blood flow, and it reduces your risk of some of this country's biggest killer diseases, including heart attacks, strokes, and diabetes. As I've said repeatedly, those health conditions also happen to be well-known contributors to cognitive decline. A number of recent studies have been aimed at discovering whether physical activity might protect against cognitive deterioration, too. Many have concluded that such a protective effect does indeed exist. Is that because exercise decreases your chance of stroke, or for another reason? Whatever the conclusion, clinical trials are now under way that will test exercise as a possible intervention against cognitive decline.

A population-based study of 1,500 people on aging and dementia in Finland found that those who engaged in leisure-time physical activity at least twice a week through middle age carried half the risk of developing dementia and a 60 percent lower risk of developing Alzheimer's compared with those who remained sedentary in their midlife. Although this relationship was seen in the entire population, the protective link was most pronounced in carriers of the APO-Eε4 allele, suggesting that exercise carries some protective factor that can impede latent Alzheimer's pathology.

In the Canadian Study of Health and Aging, a prospective community-based study of 4,600 elderly Canadians begun in the 1990s, researchers found that among women polled, the more frequent and intense the exercise reported, the lower the risk of dementia and Alzheimer's disease. A similar association was found in another study designed to learn about osteoporosis via health questionnaires given to six thousand women at six- and eight-year follow-ups. Nearly a quarter of the women who reported walking the shortest distances experienced cognitive decline, compared with only 17 percent of those who reported walking the greatest distances. Similarly, when researchers looked at the number of calories burned, the percentage of women who burned the fewest calories who went on to develop cognitive decline was higher than the percentage of women burning the most calories who went on to develop cognitive decline. Physical activity was assessed by a self-report that included such measures as distance walked and kilocalories used per week.

That means that those who walked the greatest weekly distances and ate the fewest calories had more than a one-third decrease in Alzheimer's risk compared with those who reported the least walking and greatest number of calories. Statistically, that's huge. While this relationship may seem like common sense when it comes to heart health, it is good news for those of us looking to stave off dementia and Alzheimer's disease as we grow older. Once again, the lifestyle choices we are already encouraged to make for our heart, bones, and vascular system also do good things for the brain.

In another prospective U.S. study of dementia, researchers assessed two thousand nondemented seniors in Seattle for an average of six years. Over the course of this period, 158 participants developed dementia, 107 of those developing Alzheimer's disease. After adjusting for age and gender-related risk, researchers found that people who exercised three times a week or more had an almost 40 percent risk reduction for developing Alzheimer's. The study relied on self-reporting and covered a population that had already had a relatively high proportion of regular exercisers at baseline. Nevertheless, studies of nonexercising adults have reached similar conclusions, and the link between delayed onset of dementia/Alzheimer's disease and exercise confers it with extra value in the lives of elderly people.

CASE STUDY

One Fit Lady

Beverly, a seventy-eight-year-old woman who participates in our Sun Health Brain and Body Donation Program, is an excellent example of what a person can do. She is a retired teacher who was widowed and now lives alone. She has a significant family history of Alzheimer's disease in a sister, a father, and grandparents.

She is also one of our most energetic participants. She exercises for two hundred minutes per week (mostly brisk walking), travels regularly, and is an active member of several social organizations such as Kiwanis and Rotary Club. She keeps physically fit and mentally active, both as a means of reducing her risk and improving her quality of life.

Alas, there are very few, if any, research topics in the medical community that arrive at absolute consensus, and I hazard to say we would all be a bit leery of our data if they did. So I must admit that not all studies in this area have found statistically significant links between increased exercise and Alzheimer's risk reduction.

There are several possible explanations for this inconsistency of findings. First, experts agree that the most effective exercise programs, like healthy diets, should be long-range affairs, undertaken over years and not months. Since studies must, by nature, limit their timeframes—and this is especially true when conducting large community-based studies in elderly populations—they may be unable to capture adequately the routine and results behind a long-term exercise plan. In other words, a short-term clinical trial or clinical observation study may not accurately reflect a protective benefit of an activity like exercise, since these studies are short but the protection from exercise takes years, perhaps decades, to achieve.

It is also plausible that different types of physical activity might confer different cognitive protection, so that narrowing the definition of notions such as "physical activity" and "regular" would lend greater validity to such results. For instance, these studies ought to illuminate which particular cognitive function interacts with what kind of physical exercise. The studies that have not found an association may, in fact, be inadvertently generalizing *cognitive function* but only assessing one or two measures of cognition. So we are left to define our terms and ask more questions: What kind of exercise needs to be done? How frequently should we do it? How long must your regular exercise session last for it to have any impact on your brain health?

A study by Dr. Arthur Kramer and colleagues at the University of Illinois helps illustrate just why these questions are important. After a series of tests intended to measure baseline cognitive skills, 120 nonexercising seniors between the ages of sixty and seventy-five were divided randomly into two groups. The first group was instructed to walk (aerobic exercise) and the other to do stretching and toning exercises (anaerobic). The participants were retested in six months.

Researchers found improved performance on tasks requiring greater executive (planning, task sorting) control among members of the aerobic group, but not in the anaerobic group. For tasks less dependent on executive control, no differences in cognitive performance between the aerobic and anaerobic groups were found.

Studies also seem to indicate that it is not just how often you exercise; the duration and the type of exercise matters just as much. A review of eighteen long-term studies on exercise and dementia revealed that the length and breadth of the workout—that is, how many different physical activities an individual regularly engages in—affect the overall strength of the benefit to cognitive protection. In all eighteen studies, the activities were classified as either (1) aerobic exercise, (2) a combination of aerobic exercise and strength training, or (3) no exercise at all. Overall, the review found that seniors who engaged in greater physical activity (the combination of aerobic and strength training) experienced greater cognitive improvement than did those who did no exercise at all. A general comparison of the exercise groups and control groups showed that although both groups improved in cognitive function between baseline and follow-up, the combination exercise programs were more beneficial than were programs involving aerobic exercise alone. Exercise sessions of less than thirty minutes had *no statistically significant effect on cognitive functioning*, meaning that the duration of your workout must exceed a half-hour to get any potential brain benefit.

Maintaining a moderate or high level of physical activity can add years to your life, even if you have a health condition such as diabetes and heart disease. Analysis of the famous Framingham study that involved over five thousand individuals for decades found that people who engaged in moderate physical activity lived for 2.3 years longer than did their sedentary counterparts—and that those who engaged in high levels of physical activity added four or more years to their lives.

Possible Mechanisms

Scientists hope transgenic mice (mice genetically engineered to develop Alzheimer's disease) may give us clues as to how pumping iron or riding a bike might bolster our brain's ability to ward off Alzheimer's. In one study, the number of the amyloid plaques and neurofibrillary tangles that characterize Alzheimer's (as described in chapter 2) was diminished in the brains of mice provided with a running wheel for five months, as compared with the control group without running wheels. Moreover, the mice with running wheels learned new tasks better and faster than did the mice without the benefit of regular exercise. This supports scientists' theory that animals grown in stimuli-rich environments tend to learn and readjust to environmental changes more quickly.

In fact, rodents who exercise showed decreased levels of beta-amyloid protein in their brains. But really, how could exercise actually change the brain? The first possibility is that exercise may regulate processing of APP (amyloid precursor protein, chapter 2), shifting it away from producing the toxic protein. The second possibility is that exercise in animals may increase the levels of a well-known healer chemical in the brain called *brain-derived neurotrophic factor* (BDNF). These findings suggest that exercise may provide specific anti-Alzheimer's properties above and beyond simply improving circulation.

Exercise Matters to Your Gray Matter

If you don't exercise already, building thirty minutes of exercise with a cardiovascular element into your day should be a top priority. Unless you have a previous health condition that makes physical exercise an undue risk (and you should always consult your physician before beginning any training program), moderate physical activity is a veritable wonder drug for heart health, blood flow, stroke prevention, and body weight, with great side effects that include muscle tone and mood improvement. Now many scientists are adding brainpower to that list—and the science for this is only getting stronger. Seems we should, too.

Easy Exercises for Maximum Benefits
(at least 30 minutes daily)

- Brisk walking (a treadmill works, too)
- Bicycling (stationary or two-wheel)

- Running/jogging
- Swimming
- Aerobics
- Dancing (briskly)
- Martial arts (without injuring yourself)
- Step/elliptical trainer

Final Thoughts and Recommendations

- "Maintain your brain" (see the Alzheimer's Association' Web site, www.alz.org).
- Stay physically active: walk or do other moderate repetitive exercise for at least thirty minutes daily. Aerobic activity appears to be better in this regard. Supplementing this activity with strength training is even better for the brain.
- Set real targets. Think of exercise as taking medication. Work toward a goal of aerobic exercise for thirty minutes daily. A sustained exercise program done regularly is better than intense exercise done infrequently
- Most studies examining a link between exercise and Alzheimer's show decreased risk of developing Alzheimer's in those who exercise.
- Exercise reduced Alzheimer's changes in the brains of mice that have been genetically engineered to develop the disease.

15

Staying Sharp with Mental Exercises

Our genes certainly contribute to the development of Alzheimer's, but so do the choices we make. A powerful deterrent to cognitive decline may be vigorous mental activity. There is emerging evidence that leisure activities and, in particular, cognitively stimulating activities, may be a step in the right direction when it comes to Alzheimer's prevention. Such activities have recently been reported to reduce the risk of Alzheimer's disease and are associated with a slower rate of cognitive decline.

Flexing Your Mind Muscles

In one recent study, researchers analyzed twenty years of data from almost five hundred elderly adults enrolled in the Bronx Aging Study. Over those two decades, one in four developed dementia. Among those who did not suffer from dementia and who had higher scores on cognitive exams and other measures of brain health, researchers saw that many of them cited their interest in board games, playing a musical instrument, doing puzzles, and reading. In that study, dancing was the only physical activity associated with a lower risk of dementia. The effect was dose-dependent, meaning that the likelihood of developing dementia was inversely proportional to the amount of mental and social activity engaged in. The subjects in the highest third—those who participated in the most mentally engaging activities—were 54 percent less likely to develop mild cognitive impairment (MCI) (pre-Alzheimer's, described in chapter 1) than were those in the lowest third.

Diplomas and Dementia: The Education Connection

Numerous studies, including one published in 2006, have shown a consistent link between the level of education and dementia/ cognitive decline. It appears that the more education a person has, the less likely she or he is to develop dementia. Alternatively, per-haps a lower level of education merely shifts the onset of demen-tia to an earlier stage of life, rather than increasing the risk of dementia in the first place. Education is not a sure-fire preventa-tive, however. Once the symptoms of Alzheimer's disease have appeared, if other factors stack up to cause the disease, cognitive decline is more rapid among the more highly educated.

Like so much of the literature on dementia, the links between education and dementia risk are intricate and complex. It is pos-sible that highly educated people are less likely to develop Alzheimer's for reasons that may or may not be directly associated with their education level. The "cognitive reserve theory" proposes that education leads to increased numbers of connections between brain cells and that this network of connections leads to increased intellectual function. These neural networks are required for pur-suing advanced studies. Problem solving and analysis of large amounts of data are skills attained with a rigorous education and are maintained by the professions that follow them. The idea is that once a rich and complex network of connections is forged and sustained between brain cells, such networks can stave off damage from the pathology of dementia that accumulates in the brain with age. The existence of such intricate connections means that a considerable amount of tissue destruction must take place before the system is compromised and disease becomes clinically evident. Thus, despite the seeming protective effect of education, the net result means that once Alzheimer's disease progresses far enough to be diagnosed in a highly educated person, more damage has accumulated. The subsequent decline into dementia then appears to occur at a much faster rate.

In support of the cognitive reserve theory championed by Dr. David Snowdon of the University of Kentucky, a group of nuns in the American Midwest were examined for decades while they were alive and followed to autopsy. When their brains were examined at autopsy, many of the nuns (especially the ones who were more educated and intellectually engaged) who had shown no demonstrable cognitive decline during life had enough Alzheimer's changes in their brains to fulfill a diagnosis of Alzheimer's. Dr. Snowdon attributed this disconnect to the high level of cognitive activity in which the nuns engaged, such as reading, writing, and teaching. Dr. David A. Bennett and colleagues at Rush University in Chicago performed autopsies on clergy who participated in the Religious Orders Study. These researchers at Rush University found that more educated clergy who had amounts of Alzheimer's pathology similar to those in less educated clergy showed less cognitive impairment during life. Again, this suggests that Alzheimer's damage is better tolerated in the brains of those with the higher levels of cognitive function and activity associated with education.

Researchers at Columbia University in New York set out to assess the relationship between education and rates of decline in Alzheimer's. During the course of a community-based multiethnic study of several thousand New York residents who were sixty-five years of age, 312 patients were diagnosed with Alzheimer's and were followed for an average of almost six years. Participants received periodic cognitive tests, and those with greater degrees of education demonstrated proportionally accelerated cognitive decline. "The researchers concluded that higher-educated Alzheimer's patients experience faster cognitive decline." This seems to confirm investigators' hypothesis that more highly educated individuals have accumulated more disease burden in their brains and there comes a point when they can no longer compensate for these deficits. Overall, the studies suggest that while higher educational attainment protects against developing Alzheimer's to begin with, it seems to not protect or, even worse, it seems to act against people once they have developed Alzheimer's.

The alternative explanation is that the perceived protective effect from education is actually a function of higher intelligence. In a paper published in a leading geriatrics journal, researchers obtained information from high school records of four hundred elderly people and found that the higher the IQ scores and longer the list of school activities, the lower the rates of Alzheimer's disease. Every standard deviation in IQ—about a ten-point increase—decreased the risk for dementia and MCI by 50 percent. Further, this study found that people who participated in two or more intellectually engaging activities per year were 67 percent less likely to develop Alzheimer's than were those who participated in no such activities.

Yet another study in Cleveland measured the midlife mental activity of 193 Alzheimer's victims and 358 nondemented individuals and assessed this association with the later development of Alzheimer's. Researchers gathered data on twenty-six nonoccupational activities (such as playing musical instruments, volunteering, reading, writing, pursuing artistic activities, and so forth) that participants were likely to have performed in early adulthood (twenties and thirties) and middle adulthood (forties and fifties). Individuals who did not develop Alzheimer's later in life reported having participated in more of these early activities than those who did experience symptoms of the disease. On average, these nondemented individuals spent more hours devoted to intellectual activities (reading, writing, and learning) than did those who eventually developed Alzheimer's. Study subjects who increased their intellectual activities as they moved from early to middle adulthood were also more likely to be in the nondemented group, leading investigators to speculate that participation in cognitive activities—long before dementia sets in—may increase cognitive reserve.

One of the best ways to ascertain the relevance of a certain risk or a certain protective behavior is to study genetically identical twins, because it allows scientists to assess how different environmental factors play out on identical genetic playing fields. One twenty-year study examined 107 same-sex pairs of twins in which one twin had been diagnosed as having dementia but the individual's brother (or sister) had not. The researchers assessed how often and how long each twin engaged in mentally stimulating activities. Twins who participated in a greater variety of activities had a lower risk of dementia, although this was more apparent among female twins than male ones. Although the initial assessment of leisure activity participation occurred more than twenty years prior to a dementia diagnosis, it also means that early dementia symptoms were less likely to have caused an individual's withdrawal from leisure activity.

Yet another study, the Active Study Group, a research study measuring activity levels of elderly adults, divided more than 2,800 individuals between the ages of sixty-five and ninety-four into four groups. Three of the groups received training in memory, reasoning, or speed processing, while the fourth group was given no such training. The cognitive function in the groups who received training improved, but only in speed processing. Despite encouraging results, there is not much evidence at this time that "memory training" as an isolated activity improves overall cognitive function or can delay the onset of dementia.

Most of these studies have been done in Western Europe and the United States on predominantly Caucasian populations, but data supporting a protective effect against cognitive decline in a non-Caucasian population have recently come out of China. The Chongqing Aging Study is a population-based, longitudinal study of 5,437 Chinese urban community residents older than fifty-five. Subjects were interviewed about their frequency of participation in six cognitive activities, four physical activities, two social activities from which composite scores were derived, and watching television. Each one-point increase on the cognitive score was associated with approximately a 5 percent lower risk of developing cognitive impairment. The result was mostly due to playing board games (primarily mahjong, a traditional Chinese board game) and reading. Neither the physical nor the social activity score was related to cognitive impairment.

Interestingly, watching television was associated with approximately a 20 percent *increased* risk of developing cognitive impairment. These associations were robust and remained significant after adjusting for comorbidities (meaning other medical conditions) and after excluding people who developed cognitive impairment during the first follow-up year.

Together, these studies add support to data suggesting that a modification to lifestyle, namely the frequency with which people engage in cognitively stimulating activities, may lower the risk of cognitive impairment in old age. The net sum of the information gathered is that sustained, fully engaged mental activity makes the brain more resistant to later decline. It may turn out to be one of the strongest protections against brain aging.

What We Don't Know

The mechanism by which certain mental activities seem to be protective is still somewhat of a mystery. It is possible that

---

Which Activities Might Maintain Brain Health?

- Social stimulation: traveling, volunteering, social clubs
- Mental activity: board games, crossword puzzles, creating art, adult education courses, reading, writing, learning new languages, card games, mahjong, sudoku, playing musical instruments, and crafts requiring intellectual skills and close attention such as knitting and quilting (as these require arithmetic, geometry, and memory).

individuals who engage in active lifestyles may also engage in other health and dietary behaviors with positive health benefits.

A growing body of circumstantial evidence supports the theory that education and other stimulating cognitive activities somehow confer protection against the symptoms of MCI or Alzheimer's by building up a "cognitive reserve" that in effect helps the brain ward off damage by Alzheimer's pathology.

One such study put groups of rats in two separate environments. One group of rats was kept in an enriched environment (containing toys, wheels, and other objects). The other group of rats did not have these available. The rats raised in the enriched environment were found to have a higher density of synaptic connections (connections between brain cells) than did the animals that did not have the enriched environment. But while the notion of cognitive reserve theory is attractive and intuitive, hard scientific evidence to support it as a neurological mechanism has not surfaced.

Traditional thinking about brain development and cognitive function held that the brain was static, unable to form new brain cells or replace expired ones. But there is now emerging evidence that neurogenesis—the brain's ability to regenerate and heal—occurs even late in the human life span, perhaps through growing synaptic density.

But like much Alzheimer's and dementia research, big causal questions remain largely unanswered. For instance, does engaging in mental and social activities, such as attending classes, playing a musical instrument, or doing the *New York Times* crossword every Friday, help prevent the development of dementia and keep cognitive function high? Or do those with preexisting high cognitive function or intelligence choose to engage in these activities in old age, whereas those in the subclinical stages of dementia self-select away from such cognitively challenging activities, withdrawing as a conscious or unconscious response to the onset of cognitive impairment? Both explanations are possible, even likely.

What You Can Do

Even without having sorted the chickens from the eggs, most experts agree that encouraging people to engage in fulfilling activities in their community or to trade the remote for a board game or deck of cards in hopes it might confer some cognitive protection is a bet worth making. The potential benefit for your brain and body isn't counteracted by undue risks, and compared to the skyrocketing prices at the pharmacy, the cost of dancing, reading, working on the computer, or playing Yahtzee, chess, Scrabble, or other board games is modest. Or if these "prescriptions" sound too much like drudgery, videogame makers are offering new options for seniors to get their dose of mental activity the way their kids and grandkids do. Researchers are positive that Nintendo's "Brain Age" and other puzzle games geared to older people are a fun formula for reaping the benefits of cognitive activity. Researchers are continuing to build studies that ask new questions and try to tease out the relationship between mental exercise and Alzheimer's. But in the meantime, consider renewing your library card or filling your prescription with sudoku. Or hogging your grandson's video games—just be sure to tell him it's for your health.

CASE STUDY

Mental Activity or Just Plain Good Luck?

Lucille, another of our participants in the brain donation program at Sun Health Research Institute, is eighty-one years old and a resident of Sun City. Despite having a significant family history of Alzheimer's, she is one of the most energetic and dynamic participants I know. She participates in as many research studies as her busy schedule allows. In addition to playing bridge weekly and being a voracious reader, this woman also holds leadership roles in several regional women's associations.

Despite the risk factors stacked against Lucille—age, gender, family history—she is cognitively normal. Is it just good luck or the constant mental stimulation of the life she leads?

Final Thoughts and Recommendations

- "Maintain your brain" (Alzheimer's Association, www.alz .org).
- Stay mentally active through mentally stimulating activities such as board games, crossword puzzles, creating art, adult education courses, reading, writing, learning new languages, card games, mahjong, sudoku, and playing musical instruments. This may be even more important than physical activity. Take a course at a community college. Go to the library. Learn to use a computer (Most public libraries offer free use of on-site computers for Internet access and word processing, so price is no object.)
- Make learning a lifelong project.
- Think of engaging in stimulating mental activity as akin to taking medication.

16

Anti-inflammatories and Alzheimer's

Have you ever taken an anti-inflammatory for your aches and pains, perhaps for arthritis or a headache? Interestingly, some of those medications that help your joint pain may help your brain, too. In this chapter, I explore the link between taking anti-inflammatories on a regular basis and the risk of developing Alzheimer's.

What We Know

As I discussed in earlier chapters, examination of autopsy brains from Alzheimer's patients has shown consistent inflammatory damage. Inflammation is a body's response to injury. It can cause swelling and can occur in almost any part of the body. Inflammation is considered a normal physiological response but sometimes it can amplify damage already done. Inflammation occurs in a variety of conditions including arthritis and other rheumatological conditions, and neurological diseases such as multiple sclerosis. Recently, it has been implicated in cardiovascular disease, as well.

In the medical community, it is widely held that inflammation is likely to compound, if not cause, the core pathological changes that occur in the Alzheimer's-affected brain. The thinking is that beta-amyloid protein is not welcome in the brain, so brain cells called glia and microglia try to remove this protein. They secrete a lot of chemicals including complement, cytokines, and interleukins that promote the inflammatory response. These findings occurred two decades ago, as one of the first discoveries toward understanding the biology of Alzheimer's disease. That understanding led to the premise that anti-inflammatory medication could be used to treat Alzheimer's. But first, let's talk about anti-inflammatories in a more general sense.

What Are NSAIDs?

Anti-inflammatories are also known as NSAIDS (nonsteroidal anti-inflammatory drugs). NSAIDs are used to treat a variety of conditions, including fever, arthritis, joint pain, back pain, and inflammation. They are used acutely (short-term for sudden, temporary problems such as sprains and breaks) or chronically (for ongoing conditions such as rheumatoid arthritis).

There are several medications included in this category: ibuprofen (Advil, Motrin), naproxen (Aleve, Anaprox, Naprosyn, Naprelan, and generic brands), flurbiprofen (Ansaid), diclofenac (Voltaren, Arthrotec, Cataflam), indomethacin (Indocin), celecoxib (Celebrex), sulfasalazine (Azulfidine), oxaprozin (Daypro), salsalate (Disalcid), diflunisal (Dolobid), keterolac (Toradol), etodolac (Lodine), meloxicam (Mobic), ketoprofen (Oruvail), and nabumetone (Relafen). The original anti-inflammatory is, of course, aspirin. Aspirin, however, better serves as a blood thinner to lower heart attack and stroke risk than other NSAIDs. It has negligible brain effects. Most are available by prescription. Both ibuprofen and naproxen are available in over-the-counter and prescription forms. Some NSAIDs, such as rofecoxib (Vioxx) or valdecoxib (Bextra) are no longer available due to adverse medical complications. Keep in mind that even "safe" NSAIDs can damage the kidneys and stomach if taken for prolonged periods of time. Chronic use of NSAIDs is a leading cause of stomach ulcers. Use them with care.

NSAIDs and the Link to Alzheimer's Disease

NSAIDs once got significant attention when they showed evidence that they may be useful in preventing or treating Alzheimer's. Large, population-based studies have consistently demonstrated an association between NSAID use and subsequent decreased risk of developing Alzheimer's. Using data from the Rotterdam study, investigators identified an association between a lower risk of Alzheimer's and the use of NSAIDs when taken for at least two years. The Cache County Study group reported similar findings in 2002: those who reported having taken NSAIDs for more than two years were at a lower risk of developing Alzheimer's. The same preventive association did not hold for those currently taking NSAIDs.

In surveys of the literature, more than twenty-five of these epidemiological (large, population-based) studies suggest that prior exposure to certain NSAIDs decreases the risk of Alzheimer's, delays dementia onset, slows progression of the disease, and reduces the severity of cognitive symptoms. In such meta-studies (a study of studies), consumption of anti-inflammatories on an ongoing basis resulted in a 50 percent risk reduction for Alzheimer's. And in 2004, a genetic study showed that people taking NSAIDs were 36 percent less likely to develop Alzheimer's than were family members not taking anti-inflammatories; this was especially true of those with the APO-Eε4 gene. Importantly, however, a majority of studies surveyed found no benefit or an increased Alzheimer's risk when NSAIDs were taken within two years of dementia onset, suggesting that the timing of anti-inflammatory exposure may be critical to its effect.

This wave of epidemiological evidence led to significant interest in the use of NSAIDs to treat Alzheimer's, and several medications have been investigated, including indomethacin (Indocin), diclofenac/misoprostol (Arthrotec), rofecoxib (Vioxx), and prednisone.

But the medical community's optimism about NSAIDs as Alzheimer's fighters has been tempered by the fact that clinical trials of rofecoxib, naproxen, nimesulide, and diclofenac showed *no* benefit in the treatment of Alzheimer's or mild cognitive impairment. Rofecoxib may have even accelerated cognitive decline in two of the trials. It may be that a significantly longer treatment period may be needed to show any positive results of the drugs.

Possible Mechanisms

Considerable laboratory evidence suggests that NSAIDs could protect against Alzheimer's. For instance, cyclooxygenase-2 inhibitors, commonly called *COX-2 inhibitors* (such as celecoxib, sold as Celebrex) suppress activation of microglia, the brain cells that support the neurons. Like so much of our bodies' biochemical and cellular makeup, microglia also perform helpful functions. They are actually programmed to chew up amyloid and can always be found in the vicinity of the plaques that harbor it. But in these plaque regions, the microglia release cytokines, which can compound cellular and inflammatory damage by

- Stimulating programmed cell death (apopstosis)
- Promoting amyloid accumulation and plaque formation
- Inhibiting neuronal healing in the hippocampus (where memory is stored)
- Overstimulating brain cells (excitotoxicity)

So COX-2 inhibitors could help minimize this damage by suppressing the inflammatory chain set off by the trigger-happy microglia.

Several specific anti-inflammatories seem to have additional anti-Alzheimer's effects. Ibuprofen, indomethacin, diclofenac, fenoprofen, meclofenamate, piroxicam, sulindac, and flurbiprofen (which is not yet available in the United States) may actually reduce Alzheimer's changes in the brain by reducing the effect of an enzyme called *gamma-secretase* (see chapter 2). Gamma-secretase is one of two enzymes responsible for production of beta-amyloid, the building block of brain plaque.

Certain anti-inflammatory–type medications have specific anti-Alzheimer's effects, a fact not lost on the biotech and pharmaceutical industry. Myriad Pharmaceuticals, in Salt Lake City, Utah, is developing a variant of the NSAID R-flurbiprofen, designed with Alzheimer's prevention in mind. R-flurbiprofens work by modifying gamma-secretase without the adverse effects on the stomach or kidneys seen in some other classes of NSAIDs.

Myriad is presently engaged in Phase III clinical trials designed to examine the effect of higher doses of the drug on mildly affected participants, and news from the first two phases in the United States and Great Britain was good. If these clinical trials succeed, R-flurbiprofen therapy could be on the market as a new Alzheimer's treatment by late 2008 or early 2009. Stay tuned.

What We Don't Know

Clinical trials that have investigated the use of NSAIDs for the treatment of Alzheimer's do not address the potential for Alzheimer's *prevention*. The Alzheimer's Disease Anti-inflammatory Prevention Trial (ADAPT) was designed to do just that—test the effectiveness of certain NSAIDs as a prevention strategy. Sun Health Research Institute was a participating site. Starting in January 2001, 2,500 participants at least seventy years old with at least one first-degree relative (mother, father, sister, or brother) who had Alzheimer's were enrolled in the program and have been followed ever since. These individuals were assigned to one of three treatment groups: high-dose celecoxib, high-dose naproxen, or a placebo.

In December 2004, the ADAPT study officers and senior investigators voted to suspend treatment in the trial owing, in part, to safety concerns that had been announced that winter concerning rofecoxib. Although this drug was not one of the NSAIDs being used in ADAPT, participants expressed concern about continuing to take its cousin, celecoxib. ADAPT was being conducted to test the hypothesis that celecoxib or naproxen reduces the incidence of Alzheimer's; however, preliminary results indicated no such effect, at least over the brief period of observation in the study. At this point, we can say at least that naproxen and celecoxib do not protect against developing Alzheimer's in advanced age or immediately prior to onset of memory loss.

What is still unclear at this point is whether one particular NSAID (ibuprofen, indomethacin, diclofenac, fenoprofen, meclofenamate, piroxicam, sulindac, and flurbiprofen) is more protective than another. For example, the dose needed to get a gamma-secretase–modulating effect from ibuprofen is 2,400 mg a day. Also, if NSAIDS are an effective preventative, we are still unprepared to prescribe a duration or dosage that would maximize potential dementia benefits at the risk of causing gastrointestinal damage. All of the studies suggest that NSAIDs need to be taken for long periods of time and should be taken several years before onset of symptoms in much the same way that aspirin is prescribed for those who want to prevent heart disease. And, to date, NSAIDS are not effective once Alzheimer's has taken hold in the brain. Even two years before the onset of symptoms, the potential protective value of NSAIDs has disappeared.

To answer these questions, extensive clinical trials, like the one in the works at ADAPT still need to be undertaken. Getting funding and participants for such trials may prove challenging, as drug companies don't stand to profit from any discoveries made about old, unpatented NSAIDs, and the public remains rightly concerned about the safety of certain classes of anti-inflammatory drugs.

What You Can Do

The bottom line with NSAIDs: proceed with caution. All of these medications have significant damaging effects on the kidney and the stomach if taken at high doses for long periods of time (months through years). As noted, NSAIDs are the most common cause of stomach ulcers. It is likely that long before you prevent Alzheimer's by taking these medications, you might cause irreparable harm to your stomach or kidneys. Additionally, the ADAPT study found that there is a modest but significant increased risk of stroke or heart attack for those taking naproxen for long periods of time, although a similar risk was not found with celecoxib (Celebrex).

Since not all NSAIDs appear to be the same, consider ibuprofen, indomethacin, diclofenac, fenoprofen, meclofenamate, piroxicam, sulindac, and flurbiprofen as a potential short-term treatment when NSAIDs are appropriate for a non-Alzheimer's-related condition. That way, you take care of your immediate ailment (for example, arthritis pain) and maybe help your brain in the process.

Mostly, continue any pain treatment program you've made with your doctor, but be sure to consult him or her before you make any changes regarding anti-inflammatory medications.

Final Thoughts and Recommendations

- Inflammation is a recognizable change in the brains of people suffering from Alzheimer's and likely contributes to the damage that occurs in the disease.

- Long-term consumption of anti-inflammatory medications may reduce Alzheimer's risk over time, but newer studies suggest that taking these medications within two years of onset of symptoms does not protect against developing Alzheimer's and may even have negative effects.

- Anti-inflammatory medications do not appear to be useful as treatment for Alzheimer's once symptoms have started.

- Certain anti-inflammatories—ibuprofen, indomethacin, diclofenac, fenoprofen, meclofenamate, piroxicam, sulindac, and flurbiprofen—may have specific anti-Alzheimer's properties.

- Do not use these anti-inflammatories indefinitely or in high dosage because they can damage your kidneys and stomach. Some may even increase your risk of stroke or heart attack.

- You should discuss with your physician the risks of taking anti-inflammatory medication for any length of time.

17

Vitamins May Protect

Over the years, vitamin consumption has garnered a lot of attention in the medical press and the public sphere. Store shelves are fully stocked with whole alphabets of vitamins, and millions of these bottles find their way to the medicine cabinets of Americans in hopes that they might help stave off horrible diseases such as Alzheimer's and cancer. Another reason vitamins are so commonly consumed is the feeling that it is a concrete step toward wellness that can be taken by individuals who may be unwilling to overhaul their diets, lifestyle, or health habits. Indeed, there are many reports about the general positive benefits of taking vitamins even when specific benefits are not substantiated by rigorous clinical or scientific studies. The wellness industry, spearheaded by the daily consumption of vitamins, is a $16 billion industry. It is anticipated that the wellness industry could top $1 trillion in the next decade as consumers embrace the idea of disease prevention and health promotion more and more.

In that context, it would be ideal if vitamins were a cornerstone of Alzheimer's prevention. Many vitamins have been studied with an eye toward Alzheimer's prevention and treatment. The most studied of these vitamins for Alzheimer's are the B vitamins, vitamin C, and vitamin E, although much work still remains to determine how and if these or other vitamins might contribute to cognitive health. Right now, I will put forward what we know and what we don't.

The B Vitamins (B_1, B_3, B_5, B_6, and B_{12}) and Folic Acid

The B-complex vitamins—B_1, B_3, B_5, B_6, and B_{12}—are essential for nervous system function. In supplement form, vitamin B combinations have been shown to boost certain aspects of cognitive function. Folic acid is frequently formulated with these vitamins and has its own protective qualities. B vitamins are water soluble, meaning that the body tends to clear them through the urine. They are unlikely to reach toxic levels because they are not stored in large amounts in the body.

Recommendations in This Chapter and from the RDA

The FDA publishes *recommended daily allowances* (called the RDA) for vitamins. These are guidelines that are meant to ensure proper nutrition and prevent nutritional deficiencies. The RDAs are found on every bottle of vitamins and almost every cereal box. Keep in mind that vitamins are also found in food sources. Many food items are enriched with vitamins, and still many more, such as dark, leafy vegetables, naturally contain significant amounts of vitamins. In fact, dietary consumption is the most common way to take in vitamins. In this chapter, I make recommendations for consumption of specific vitamins in specific quantities. Most of the recommendations I make exceed the RDA and should not be confused with the RDA. Nevertheless, the doses recommended have been shown to be generally safe.

B$_1$

Vitamin B$_1$, or thiamine, is directly involved in brain metabolic functions, and can help with reaction time and mental energy. A sudden deficiency of thiamine, most often caused by heavy alcohol consumption, can cause confusion, vision problems, and difficulties with balance and walking (in medical parlance, this triad is called Wernicke's encephalopathy). When the lack of thiamine becomes a chronic deficiency, a dementia emerges (called Korsakoff dementia; see chapter 12). The recommended dose is 50 mg daily for cognitive health.

B$_3$

B$_3$, or niacin, is an important B vitamin in glucose metabolism, and has been shown to increase blood flow and lower cholesterol. We know that severe niacin deficiency can cause dementia, but recently researchers wondered whether dietary levels of niacin might have some effect on age-related neurodegeneration or the development of Alzheimer's. Over the course of the Chicago Health and Aging Project, clinical evaluations and food frequency questionnaires helped researchers look for links between if/when participants developed Alzheimer's or cognitive decline, and the niacin levels in their food and supplement intake.

The investigators did find a protective link between amount of niacin consumed and cognitive health: participants with the highest niacin intake levels were less likely to develop Alzheimer's over

---

Units of Measure

We are talking tiny here.

Vitamins are usually measured in milligrams, micrograms, or international units. 1 microgram is 1/1000th of a milligram or 1/1,000,000th of a gram. An international unit is basically a standard set by the scientific community.

the course of the study than were those with the lowest niacin intake, and a higher niacin food intake was connected with slower overall cognitive decline. The recommended dose is 20 mg daily.

B$_5$

B$_5$, or pantothenic acid, is an essential B vitamin for sustaining life. It is critical for the production of carbohydrates, fats, and proteins. In the brain, vitamin B$_5$ plays a role in the production of acetylcholine, a crucial neurotransmitter involved in learning and memory and the one that is lost in Alzheimer's disease. The recommended dosage for B$_5$ is 5 mg or greater daily.

B$_6$

B$_6$, or pyridoxine, assists in the balancing of chemicals such as sodium and potassium. In the brain, it is required for the production of important neurotransmitters, including serotonin, dopamine, noradrenaline, and adrenaline. The typical recommended dose is 25 to 50 mg. Exceeding 100 mg is not a good idea, since it can cause nerve damage in the feet (peripheral neuropathy).

B$_{12}$

B$_{12}$, or cyanocobolamin, is the most essential vitamin for neuronal health. It helps build the coating, or myelin sheaths, around nerve cells. Vitamin B$_{12}$ deficiencies have been closely linked with spinal cord and nerve damage, memory loss, and dementia. Treatment with high-dose B vitamins has been shown to protect against heart attacks, strokes, and death. A population-based study published in *Stroke* in 2005 showed that people who took the highest dose administered of B$_{12}$ were significantly less likely than were other participants to suffer a stroke or heart attack, reducing the risk of stroke or death by one-fifth.

B$_{12}$ deficiencies are common among those who consume excess alcohol and the elderly; some studies estimate that between 17 to 20 percent of elderly people have vitamin B$_{12}$ deficiencies. People who undergo bariatric surgery (for weight loss, such as the gastric bypass or Lap-Band), which reduces the stomach size, often develop B_{12} deficiencies because they lose the absorption surface area of the stomach lining, where this vitamin is absorbed. When a person comes in with proprioceptive loss (loss of a sense of where their feet, legs, and joints are), increased reflexes, and trouble walking, one of the things we check for is a form of B_{12} deficiency called *subacute combined degeneration*. Low blood levels of B_{12} can cause extensive neurological damage to the brain and spinal cord. If you are in any of these at-risk groups, get your B_{12} level tested, which can be done through a simple blood test (see chapter 4).

Fortunately, B_{12} is not only easily identifiable but easy to supplement, and studies show that high-dose injection and oral therapy, often administered in 1,000 mcg injections twice a month or 1,000 mcg oral doses daily, can reverse memory loss to a certain degree. Many seniors in Sun City get their B_{12} shot periodically as a means of boosting energy and mental sharpness, even when they have normal blood levels of vitamin B_{12}.

Vitamin B_{12} is not as readily absorbed by mouth as it is by injection, but supplementation with an oral form of the vitamin does gradually raise B_{12} levels. The recommended amount for cognitive health would be 1,000 mcg daily.

Folic Acid

Folic acid, sometimes called folate, is a water-soluble vitamin that is often dispensed with vitamin B_{12} (cyanocobolamin) and other B vitamins (this is marketed as "the super B complex" or the "B50 complex" or the "B100 complex"). In the literature, folic acid is one of the few vitamins whose specific isolated total intake has been significantly associated with a lowered risk of Alzheimer's. Low folate status is associated with poor cognitive function and dementia in the elderly, whereas the literature suggests that supplement-delivered folic acid may confer some protective effect for Alzheimer's risk. In the Baltimore Longitudinal Study of Aging, participants who took folic acid at or above the RDA (400 mcg daily) had a 55 percent reduced risk of developing Alzheimer's. Another study from New York confirmed the protective effects of folic acid consumption. In that study, the group with the highest folic acid intake had a 50 percent risk reduction, compared with the group taking the lowest amount of folic acid. In the study, the highest amount of folic acid was defined as greater than 480 mcgs daily.

Scientists have studied the effects of folic acid fortification in elderly Hispanic populations to tease out the relationship between folate status and cognitive function. Among the participants who underwent detailed memory and cognitive tests, folate deficiency was very rare. Folate levels correlated highly with performance on these memory tests, even after accounting for homocysteine, vitamin B_{12}, creatinine, demographic variables, and depressive symptom scores. Investigators also found that the relative risks of cognitive impairment and dementia decreased with increasing folate concentration in blood cells.

Although it is easy to feel optimistic about taking B vitamins and folic acid, not all studies identify a benefit. Recently, the results of a two-year clinical trial published in the *New England Journal of Medicine* found that lowering homocysteine levels in elderly patients with B_6, B_{12}, and folate resulted in no appreciable cognitive improvement. For two years, the investigators studied nearly three hundred participants over sixty-five years old with high homocysteine; half were treated with the vitamin supplements and half given a placebo. The researchers found no difference between the two groups' cognitive tests given at the one- and two-year marks.

Folic acid deficiency is rare in the United States today, a fact that is attributed to the nationwide supplementation of this vitamin in grain products. Since 1998, U.S. commercially produced cereals and breads have been fortified with folic acid, a relatively simple and low-cost preventive action that has significantly reduced the prevalence of folate deficiency and hyperhomocysteinemia in the United States.

Folic acid is widely available as a single vitamin, or in multivitamins or as part of B-complex vitamins. Many brands of folic acid supplements are available in most food and drug stores. Amerisciences, Herbalife, Life Extension Foundation, Trader Joe's, and all major pharmacies carry this vitamin. Taking folic acid as part of a multivitamin is fine and is a typical means of getting it in sufficient quantity. However, my preference is to take folic acid in combination with B_{12} only. A typical folic acid dose is 400 mcg daily but, for cognitive health, 800 to 1,600 mcg is the recommended target. Taking folic acid is generally safe. It is difficult to overdose on this vitamin, but excessive consumption of B_{12} is associated with diarrhea, overproduction of red blood cells, itching, rash, headaches, and swelling, so be mindful of how much B_{12} you may pair with your folic acid.

Prescription-strength folic acid vitamins are available for people needing very high doses. Cerefolin is a branded product that contains methylfolate, the most reduced and only form of folate that crosses the blood brain barrier. Methylfolate has also been shown to be seven times more viable than folic acid at reducing homocysteine levels. Pamlab, which makes Cerefolin, has published studies showing that methylfolate was superior to folic acid to reducing homocysteine levels.

Other prescription brands include Folgard and Foltx and range from 2.2 to 5 milligrams, which contain approximately eight to twelve times the over-the-counter strength.

Possible Mechanisms for Folic Acid's Effects on Cognitive Health

As I discussed earlier, high homocysteine levels are correlated with risk for Alzheimer's and heart disease. Clinical data also support a strong association between homocysteine and dementia, wherein increased levels of homocysteine are associated with cognitive decline as well as with atrophy of the brain.

Folic acid is a proven regulator of homocysteine levels and, in supplement form, has been shown to lower blood homocysteine levels by as much as 25 percent. This may be because both folic acid and vitamin B_{12} are cofactors in the methylation/demethylation cycle. The methylation/demethylation cycle is critically important to neuronal health because it regulates levels of the toxic metabolite homocysteine, as well as numerous other functions, including gene transcription, enzymatic activity, and neurotransmission. Homocysteine levels are kept low by conversion to methionine through a reaction that requires vitamin B_{12}, or by demethylation to produce cysteine. Inhibition of folate or B_{12} uptake leads to reduced regeneration of methionine, reduced substrate for methylation reactions, and increased levels of homocysteine.

Disruption of this methylation cycle through depletion of folate or vitamin B_{12} has been associated with increased degeneration of the brain and spinal cord, as well as birth defects, such as spinal bifida (which is a failure of the spine and spinal cord to form correctly during pregnancy). And reduced folate has been directly linked to elevated homocysteine levels, beta-amyloid accumulation, and increased DNA damage in transgenic mice overexpressing APP. Folic acid deficiency and elevated homocysteine levels impair DNA repair in the hippocampal neurons (the brain cells responsible for memory) and make these cells vulnerable to amyloid toxicity, in experimental Alzheimer's models.

Folic Acid: What We Still Don't Know

In 2006, the *New England Journal of Medicine* published results from the HOPE study, which was designed to investigate the risk of B vitamin and folic acid treatment in cardiovascular disease and stroke. Investigators reported that folic acid treatment did not lower the risk of cardiovascular disease but did reduce homocysteine levels and lower the risk of stroke. High levels of vitamin B_6 were associated with an increased risk in cardiovascular events, and more research needs to be done to find out whether this is a dose-related link.

A clinical trial is under way to explore high-dose folic acid as a treatment for Alzheimer's disease. Several hundred people with Alzheimer's are assigned to receive 5 mg of folic acid or matching placebo for eighteen months to determine if the vitamin can actually slow the disease progression. Results should be available soon.

Vitamins C and E

Vitamin C, or ascorbic acid, is probably the most-consumed stand-alone vitamin on the market today, and is found in an abundance of food items, such as fruit juice, fruits, and vegetables. Championed most famously by Dr. Linus Pauling, vitamin C is many people's go-to vitamin for warding off infections and maintaining general good health. Studies have demonstrated its antioxidant, anti-atherogenic (which means it prevents buildup of blockages in arteries), anticarcinogenic (cancer-preventing), antihistamine, antiviral, and antihypertensive properties, and it is recommended by the FDA to those with iron deficiencies. Since vitamin C is a water-soluble vitamin, excess amounts are urinated out and aren't toxic to your system, although too much vitamin C can cause an upset stomach or diarrhea in some individuals.

More recently, vitamin C has been the subject of extensive investigations as it relates to cognitive aid and intelligence. A famous study of schoolchildren from kindergarten to college showed that students' IQ scores raised an average of nearly 4 points when their vitamin C intake was elevated by 50 percent through supplements.

Although some community-based studies have linked taking vitamin C with increased cognitive function, this link has not been borne out across all studies, most likely due to methodological differences. In a study published in the journal *Health Nutrition and Aging,* researchers looked at the association between vitamin C and cognitive function in 544 community-dwelling older adults aged sixty-five or older who were enrolled in both the Cardiovascular Health Study (CHS) and the CLUE II study. Three percent of the subjects had low levels of vitamin C in their blood (less than 40 mg/dL) and 15 percent had low total vitamin C intake (less than 60 mg/day). Most participants (96.7 percent) had normal cognitive function. When researchers broke down scores on cognitive function and attention tests, those in the highest quintile of vitamin C concentration in their blood had significantly better scores than those in the lowest quintile, even after adjusting for other variables. In a stratified analysis by gender, higher vitamin C intake was associated with higher MMSE scores in men, but not in women.

But in a new multicenter study out of Johns Hopkins and Utah, researchers found that among 4,740 participants, those who reported taking a nutritional supplement containing 500 to 1,000 mg of vitamin C and up to 1,000 IUs of vitamin E, something about the combination of vitamins C and E seemed to reduce risk of Alzheimer's.

Overall, these mixed results do not provide strong evidence of an association between vitamin C concentrations or intake and cognitive function, but the proven antioxidant properties of vitamin C should keep it as part of your daily multivitamin regimen. The consistent thread in these studies seems to be that RDAs are not enough to confer any protection. Indeed, the Johns Hopkins participants had to take *seven times* the recommended daily allowance of vitamin C before researchers could see a protective effect. To get maximum antioxidant value from this vitamin, take 1,500 mg daily.

Recommended Dietary Allowance:

Males: 14 to 18 years old: 75 mg daily; greater than 18 years old: 90 mg daily

Females: 14 to 18 years old: 60 mg daily; greater than 18 years old: 75 mg daily

As I've discussed throughout the book, oxidative injury has been implicated in a range of serious health conditions, including atherosclerotic heart disease and cancer. And a large body of evidence implicates such oxidative cellular damage in the brains of those with Alzheimer's disease. Antioxidants are believed to work in a number of ways. They may lessen oxidation, by inactivating oxygen free radicals, and/or they may restore at least some normal functioning to tissues damaged by oxygen free radicals.

Therefore, antioxidant vitamins have been extensively evaluated in the prevention of cancer and cardiovascular diseases. Because of their established free-radical fighting properties and cognitive-boosting power, the medical community has paid as much attention to vitamins C and E as they relate to Alzheimer's prevention. And in the lab at least, these two vitamins indeed seem to work against Alzheimer's amyloid cascade.

Vitamin E is a fat-soluble vitamin, which means that when we ingest it, it can be stored in the fat. Vitamin E is actually a mixture of a group of compounds called *tocopherols*. The predominant and most active form of vitamin E is alpha-tocopherol, although it is not the kind found in food. In the lab, vitamin E has been shown to have powerful antioxidant properties, improve endothelial cell function, and to reduce atherosclerosis as well as the multiplication of certain unwanted cell types. It can improve function of cells called endothelial cells. The standard dose in a supplement is 400 IU (international units). Doses greater than 2,000 IU may increase risk of bleeding, especially when combined with blood thinners and sometimes even with aspirin.

Despite their reputation, the evidence of vitamins C and E's possible protective power from Alzheimer's or dementia is mixed. Several studies have found a reduced risk of Alzheimer's or dementia, whereas others have not. Vitamin E levels in food and plasma were found to be inversely associated with incident Alzheimer's disease in three prospective studies, but no similar association between Alzheimer's and alpha-tocepherol, the most potent form of vitamin E and the one used in supplements, was seen.

A large study conducted in Holland with 5,500 nondemented individuals aged fifty-five and older over an average course of six years looked at consumption of vitamins and supplements. Investigators found that the risk of developing Alzheimer's went down by 18 percent in study subjects with high intakes of vitamins C and E. The protective effects were still present even after taking such influences as age, gender, smoking, weight, and education into account, and were more pronounced among smokers.

Another prospective study of older individuals in Utah found reduced risk of Alzheimer's among vitamin C and E takers as well. At baseline, taking both supplements in combination reduced the risk of having Alzheimer's by almost 80 percent. When this association was reassessed after three years, using both vitamins C and E as supplements in combination still reduced the risk of Alzheimer's by 64 percent. Taking either vitamin individually did not seem to be as protective.

In contrast to these studies, one very respected scientific group using data collected from New York City residents found no protective Alzheimer's effect with these two vitamins. Nearly one thousand randomly selected Manhattan residents aged sixty-five and older met study criteria, and of these, one quarter had Alzheimer's. The investigators found no association between participants' risk of Alzheimer's and their vitamin C and E intake, either through regular diet or supplemental use. And in the Honolulu Aging Study that I've discussed before, combined vitamin C and E use was linked to a reduced risk of vascular dementia but not to Alzheimer's.

Investigators in the Chicago Health and Aging Project (CHAP) found was that people who consumed the highest amount of vitamin E were 70 percent less likely to develop Alzheimer's than were those who consumed the lowest amount; no similar protective effect was discovered for intake of vitamin C, beta-carotene, or other dietary supplements. In a different section of the study, CHAP researchers found that vitamin E intake also was linked with a slower rate of decline in those who did develop Alzheimer's.

One challenge we face as researchers is to try to extrapolate data from population-based and survey-based studies, and then translate the information into meaningful clinical findings that we can use to help patients. Ideally, we would love to correlate population-based studies to clinical trials, but to do so would be a big mistake. Keep in mind that positive effects of a substance that have been demonstrated in population studies does not equal a prescription for a treatment or the possible impact of a therapy making use of those conclusions. *Treatment of patients who already have Alzheimer's and prevention for those who don't are not the same.*

At least one clinical trial suggested a possible benefit for the antioxidant alpha-tocopherol (vitamin E) in slowing the progression of established Alzheimer's. That study investigated very high doses of vitamin E (2,000 IU) in patients with advanced Alzheimer's. They defined the range of possible outcomes of the study as death, nursing home placement, and full-time care in the home. Participants were assigned to take either vitamin E, selegiline (a Parkinson's medication that also has antioxidants), a combination of vitamin E and selegiline, or a placebo. All participants were enrolled for two years.

Individuals taking the high doses of vitamin E (2,000 IU) delayed the endpoints by 270 days, or nine months, compared to the individuals who took placebo. That is a big difference, and one that excited the medical community. By 1997, we neurologists and clinicians caring for Alzheimer's patients were recommending 2,000 IU of alpha-tocopherol as part of the treatment of Alzheimer's.

However, times change, and so do our approaches. It may turn out that vitamin E is not the "all-protective" vitamin we had hoped it to be. Two such studies call into question whether high doses of this vitamin are a good idea for the treatment or even prevention of Alzheimer's.

A meta-analysis examined the association between vitamin E supplementation and the risk of death (what we call *mortality*). This analysis found that high doses of vitamin E may actually *increase the risk* for mortality, particularly from cardiovascular events.

This collection of findings sounded a note of caution for vitamin E supplementation as a preventative measure. It also highlighted the need for more basic and clinical research on the role of oxidative stress as a risk factor of Alzheimer's and other aging-related neurodegenerative dementias. Having garnered a lot of attention, this article may well have swung the pendulum away from advocating the taking of vitamin E.

Another study published in 2005 demonstrated that high doses of vitamin E (2,000 IU) did not slow the rate of conversion from mild cognitive impairment to Alzheimer's. And in non-Alzheimer's-related studies, long-term (up to seven years) vitamin E supplementation (400 IU) has not been shown to prevent cancer or major cardiovascular events. In the HOPE trial, vitamin E even increased the risk of congestive heart failure.

Since the population-based studies suggest that consuming vitamins C and E would be beneficial to protect against Alzheimer's, but clinical studies warn against use of vitamin E as a *treatment* for Alzheimer's, what we need is a prevention trial to assess whether it can be used safely to *prevent* Alzheimer's. For now, the recommended dose for health and prevention should not exceed 400 IU.

The good news is that this trial is under way. It is called PREADVISE (Prevention of Alzheimer's Disease by Vitamin E and Selenium) and it is a part of a bigger clinical trial called SELECT (Selenium and Vitamin E Cancer Prevention Trial). The SELECT study is actually intended to determine whether vitamin E or selenium can be used to prevent prostate cancer. As the male participants enroll, they agree to undergo a memory test on a regular basis. So stay tuned: eventually, we will know if vitamin E can protect against development of Alzheimer's in a rigorous clinical trial.

Final Thoughts and Recommendations

- Folic acid deficiency has strong links to low cognitive performance and dementia in older population.

- Taking at least 800 mcg of folic acid daily seems to have a protective cognitive effect. Supplement the daily folic acid with its companion vitamin, B_{12}, at 1,000 mcg daily. Higher folic acid intake decreases the risk of developing Alzheimer's.

- Some of the B vitamins may improve healthy neurons, but their link to Alzheimer's prevention has not been definitively established. The B vitamins and their recommended dosages are summarized within the chapter.

- Vitamin C, while linked with antioxidant and cognitive properties, has not been shown to have specific anti-Alzheimer's properties. Current recommendations are 500 mg daily. The target may be as much as 1,500 mg daily.

- Vitamin E may not be as protective as we once thought. For prevention, current recommendations should not exceed 400 IUs daily. Clinical trials are under way to reassess this vitamin as a preventive agent against Alzheimer's.

- Ask your health-care provider what vitamins are safe and appropriate for you.

18

Supplements: Real Hope or Empty Promises?

Supplements are exceedingly popular, and many people consume them with the belief and expectation that they might help or prevent a broad variety of conditions. Indeed, many supplements do have biological evidence and scientific studies supporting their use. But there are just as many studies—perhaps more—that lack any convincing data to recommend their use. Just because the FDA does not require a prescription for over-the-counter supplements does not automatically mean that they are safe or effective (remember that even herbal supplements can act like *drugs*, some of which may be allergenic or toxic, or may interact with prescribed medications).

Overall, my concern is that a lot of supplements make bold claims, claims for which there is no hard scientific data. Most of these efficacy claims come with taglines like "clinical studies prove . . .," "doctor recommended," or "scientific studies reveal . . . ." In many instances, these supplements have not been subjected to rigorous scientific scrutiny or passed the litmus test of clinical trials. For that matter, almost no (except for ginkgo biloba and DHA) supplement has been used in a clinical trial as a specific preventative agent against Alzheimer's. Others have, and have passed with what amount to scientific flying colors.

In this chapter, I review the evidence of which supplements really may benefit memory and may have protective effects in the brain and which do not appear to be supported by the weight of scientific evidence. Keep in mind that there are no expert consensus guidelines or panel opinions on the subject of supplements and Alzheimer's prevention so the recommendations forthwith reflect my critical review of the medical literature.

Supplements That Focus on Cognitive Health and Protection

- Supplements with compelling evidence of protective qualities or benefit

  Ginkgo biloba
  Omega-3 Fatty Acids (DHA)
  Curcumin
  Huperzine A
  Phosphatidylserine

- Supplements with less robust evidence of protection or benefit

  Choline
  Lecithin (phosphatidylcholine)
  DHEA
  Acetyl-L-carnitine
  DMAE
  Vinpocetine
  Grapeseed extract and quercetin
  Resveratrol

I will use this list as a guide to talk a little first about supplements with good evidence of some cognitive benefit. Then I'll discuss those whose labels or reputation outweighs what science has shown.

Supplements with Compelling Evidence of Protective Qualities or Benefits

Ideally, we would love to take a supplement that improves our memory and cognitive health or outright prevents Alzheimer's. Overshadowing the possible effects of many promising supplements is the fact that most have not undergone rigorous scientific scrutiny or passed the tests that we as physicians or scientists would deem reliable. The supplements discussed below have the best scientific data supporting their use in cognitive health.

Ginkgo Biloba

Ginkgo biloba is one of the most popular and widely studied brain supplements in the world. The extract from ginkgo tree leaves, first used in ancient Chinese medicine, is known primarily for its brain benefits, and is commonly prescribed overseas for circulatory health, since it increases blood flow. Ginkgo has also been shown to have, in varying degrees, beneficial effects on memory, concentration, and other cognitive conditions, and has been used for treating various health conditions such as vertigo, altitude sickness, tinnitus (ringing in the ears), and premenstrual syndrome (a.k.a. PMS). Ginkgo biloba is packed with blood-vessel-relaxing compounds called flavonoids. Flavonoids also boast an impressive free-radical fighting reputation (free radicals and antioxidants were discussed in chapter 11).

In a study in Pacquid, France, dietary intake of flavonoids was associated with a 50 percent cut in the risk of developing dementia over the course of five years. Another study showed that dietary consumption of flavonoids was associated with a 46 percent risk reduction for developing Alzheimer's.

In 1997, the *Journal of the American Medical Association* reported some stabilization of cognitive decline in Alzheimer's and vascular dementia patients. But in a 2002 study in the same journal, ginkgo showed no appreciable cognitive effect among nondemented subjects. A prevention trial, the Ginkgo Evaluation of

Memory Study (GEMS), is currently under way, with results expected within two to three years.

The commonly recommended dose is 60 mg twice a day with meals, in a standardized 50:1 extract capsule form. Benefits are usually seen after twelve weeks of consistent supplementation.

Omega-3 Fatty Acids

In chapter 11, I addressed the cognitive protective properties of omega-3 fatty acids, especially eicosapentaenic acid (EPA) and docosahexaenoic acid (DHA). When consumed as a part of a high fish diet, they have been linked with reduced risk of developing dementia and Alzheimer's disease, as well as with overall cognitive maintenance. Alpha-linoleic acid (ALA), the plant-derived omega-3 fatty acid, has not been shown to share the same properties as DHA and EPA, which are found in fatty fish such as salmon and mackerel. Although ALA have other important therapeutic effects, including anticancer properties and suppressing inflammation as

---

Warning! Ginkgo Biloba and Blood Thinners

When it comes to ginkgo biloba, the only major contraindication I warn patients about is a blood-thinning tendency. If you are on any blood-thinning medication at all, be sure to talk to your doctor before starting ginkgo. Here are some major guidelines:

- Ginkgo and aspirin: Fine together, as long as the aspirin does not exceed 325 mg.
- Ginkgo and Coumadin: Absolutely not! This is a dangerous combination that can lead to hemorrhage.
- Ginkgo and Plavix (or other blood thinners): Ask your doctor.
- Ginkgo and vitamin E: Fine together, as long as the vitamin E dose is less than 2,000 IU.

well as laxative and demulcent properties, ALA has not been shown to have cognitive protective effects of its omega-3 counterparts, DHA and EPA.

The real protection comes mostly from DHA. To investigate the effects of DHA on Alzheimer's changes in the brain, DHA has been fed to mice genetically engineered to develop Alzheimer's. In these mice, treatment with DHA has resulted in lower amounts of the toxic beta-amyloid protein in the brain.

However, those taking DHA as a means of protecting against Alzheimer's should be aware of the recent results of a treatment trial of DHA for Alzheimer's disease. In that study, more than two hundred people were enrolled and treated with 1,700 mg of DHA (with 600 mg of EPA) or a placebo for six months. The result of that study was that DHA did not help the people with Alzheimer's disease. A careful analysis of the data reveals that those participants in the trial who had a milder form of Alzheimer's did receive some benefit. One caveat to consider is that the study was only for six months, whereas treatment will require years to demonstrate protection. Such a clinical trial is underway sponsored by the NIH. In that clinical trial, Alzheimer's subjects will take high doses of DHA or matching placebo for 18 months. Most of the focus has been to investigate DHA as a treatment for Alzheimer's but, given the strength of the epidemiological studies for fish consumption and consumption of omega-3 fatty acids, it is an optimal product to be considered for Alzheimer's prevention.

Most formulations of omega-3 fatty acids have high amounts of EPA and ALA, and modest amounts of DHA. When choosing an omega-3 supplement, select one that has a high concentration of DHA. Your target is 1,000 to 1,500 mg of DHA daily. The FDA recommends 3 g daily, from food sources, of all omega-3 fatty acids combined.

Beware: Many formulations of omega-3 have fish as their primary source and therefore have the propensity to smell and taste like fish. Also, consuming more than the 500 mg of omega-3 fatty acids can result in bloating, upset stomach, and diarrhea.

Curcumin

Surprise! Eating curry may reduce your risk for Alzheimer's. Epidemiological studies showing that India has one of the lowest prevalence rates of Alzheimer's in the world have led some researchers to look closer at curry consumption as a possible, if unexpected, Alzheimer's-fighting tactic. Some of the information in this section was provided to me by my friend and colleague John Ringman, MD, from UCLA.

For centuries, the plant *Curcuma longa* has been used in traditional Indian medicine to treat various ailments, including acid reflux, gas, liver problems, and urinary tract infections. This plant, also known as turmeric, is a member of the ginger family, and is indigenous to South and Southeast Asia. Turmeric, the principal ingredient in curry, has interesting properties that may cause it to reduce Alzheimer's risk, including antioxidant, anti-inflammatory, and cholesterol-lowering properties (see below), all three of which combat key processes in the development of Alzheimer's changes in the brain. Components of turmeric are also currently undergoing scientific evaluation as anticancer agents, and potential treatments for HIV infection and respiratory conditions. In addition to its use for medicinal purposes, the vivid yellow spice is used as a dye and food additive.

Curcumin's marquee property is probably its antioxidant action, making it an ideal early food preservative. In fact, several laboratory experiments have shown that curcumin may have even more potent antioxidant properties than vitamin E. And its anti-inflammatory effects may be the medium through which curcumin could slow Alzheimer's pathology. Recent studies have looked especially closely at curcumin's anti-inflammatory role in comparison to NSAIDS. Indeed, investigators have demonstrated that curcumin works just like and is as strong as ibuprofen and naproxen. In another study, administration of 500 mg of curcuminoids a day for seven days reduced levels of serum cholesterol in healthy volunteers. This suggests another mechanism by which curcumin might exert beneficial effects on Alzheimer's.

In the lab, scientists have demonstrated that curcuminoids, but not vitamin E, protected cells from injury induced by beta-amyloid protein and inhibited the formation and extension of amyloid fibrils in transgenic mice. By doing so, curcumin inhibits the amyloid cascade that distinguishes Alzheimer's pathology.

All these properties and its good safety profile have made curcumin a top candidate compound in the search for Alzheimer's preventive agents. But laboratory studies with mice revealed interesting complications. In a six-month curcumin study in transgenic mice carrying the Alzheimer's-tripping amyloid precursor protein, mice were fed diets containing either no curcumin, low-dose curcumin, or high-dose curcumin. The mice fed low-dose curcumin had significantly reduced levels of soluble and insoluble beta-amyloid protein as well as reduced amyloid plaque burden. In other words, they had both less Alzheimer's changes and less damage from those changes that had already accumulated. The high-dose group did as well as but not better than the low-dose group.

In another study where the amyloid was injected directly into the brains of mice, high doses of curcumin acted like an anti-inflammatory and resulted in reduction of oxidative damage and preservation of the connections between the cells called synapses. In fact, this protective effect was more robust than that seen with the anti-inflammatory ibuprofen.

Animals can be tested to determine if the protective effects of compounds such as curcumin result in beneficial effects on memory. Scientists have tested rats and mice to determine if curcumin improved memory in a water maze. Rats fed with high doses of curcumin learned to find the hidden platform in the water maze test more quickly. These findings provide evidence that curcumin can counteract the pathology and cognitive deficits in mice that get Alzheimer's, but for now leaves the actual mechanism for this activity open to question and further investigation.

Does eating curcumin really affect what goes on in the human brain? It has to get into the brain to have a protective effect, right? These are important questions that researchers are working through right now. Researchers at UCLA have performed studies that demonstrate that curcumin crosses into the brain and binds to amyloid plaques. This may be important in its antiamyloid activity. Because animal studies suggest multiple mechanisms by which curcumin might work against Alzheimer's pathology, further study of this compound in the treatment or prevention of Alzheimer's in humans is warranted.

Turmeric is currently listed as a coloring and flavoring agent in food by the Food and Drug Administration, and is widely used as such without known adverse effects. Currently the temporary acceptable daily intake level of curcumin is 0.1 mg/kg of body weight, but several short-term studies looking at the safety and tolerability of high doses have shown that doses up to 1,200 mg/day were well-tolerated in patients with rheumatoid arthritis, postsurgical patients, and ophthalmology patients. Very high doses are associated with adverse effects such as gastric irritation or nausea.

To date, no long-term safety and tolerability studies have been done on human subjects. No ideal dosage has been established, nor has been the duration needed to exert curcumin's Alzheimer's-prevention qualities. Presently, clinical trials are ongoing to investigate whether curcumin is an effective treatment for Alzheimer's patients. Current doses being investigated are 400 to 800 mg in a capsule form, and that would be the target dose for consuming curcumin on a regular basis. Like many supplements and dietary changes, it is likely that years of consumption are required for potential protective qualities to emerge.

Huperzine A

Huperzine A is an alkaloid extract of the plant *Huperzia serrata*. It is a component of a traditional Chinese herbal medicine, Qian Ceng Ta, used to treat fever and inflammation. During the 1980s, scientists in China determined that huperzine A is a potent inhibitor of the enzyme acetylcholinesterase (AChE). Remember in Alzheimer's, acetylcholine is lost because it is not being produced, as the cells that produce it are gradually dying. The enzyme responsible for breaking down acetylcholine is AChE. Inhibitors of AChE constitute the mainstay of treatment in Alzheimer's. They include donepezil (Aricept), rivastigmine (Exelon), galantamine

(Razadyne), and tacrine (Cognex). These medications are covered in more detail in chapter 19.

Huperzine, like the AChE inhibitors tacrine and donepezil, preserves acetylcholine levels in the brain. Huperzine A is now used in China to treat Alzheimer's.

Physicians and researchers in the United States are curious to know whether huperzine supplements might offer similar symptomatic relief of Alzheimer's. In addition, huperzine has antioxidant and neuroprotective properties that make it a compound of interest to the Alzheimer's community.

Several clinical trials in dementia and Alzheimer's patients in China have shown enhancement of memory and cognitive functions. In one study of 160 subjects with dementia or memory disorders, a 50 mcg dosage of huperzine A, injected twice daily for four weeks, resulted in significant improvement on memory testing, compared with saline injections. In a second study, twenty-eight Alzheimer's subjects were treated with a 200 mcg dosage of huperzine A by mouth, twice daily for sixty days. These patients showed improvement on memory testing, compared with subjects treated with a placebo. More recently, in a clinical trial of 103 subjects with Alzheimer's, treatment with a 200 mcg dosage of huperzine A, by mouth twice daily for eight weeks, was associated with significant improvement on a memory quotient, compared with placebo treatment.

Another recent Chinese study suggests that huperzine A treatment for Alzheimer's compares favorably with donepezil, rivastigmine, and galantamine in terms of cognitive benefit, as measured by the standard memory tests used in clinical trials. Because of the strength of the data, a clinical trial of this supplement is ongoing. All trials performed to date have looked at huperzine A as a treatment for, not a preventative against, Alzheimer's. That said, it has potent biological properties that make it worthy of consideration in the area of prevention.

Taking huperzine A is associated with mild side effects (primarily dizziness, nausea, and diarrhea). When side effects occur, they generally diminish with time despite continuation of treatment. No adverse effects on vital signs (blood pressure, pulse, etc.), blood tests, or electrocardiograms have been seen. The recommended daily dose is 200 to 400 mcg.

Another Chinese herbal extract being looked at for possible dementia-fighting power is called GETO, made of ginseng, epimedium herb, and thinleaf milkwort root. This compound was shown to have mild beneficial effects, compared with piracetam and a placebo, in a clinical trial of seventy elderly Chinese patients with MCI, and the authors recommend further clinical trials on this compound.

Phosphatidylserine (PS)

Phosphatidylserine is a component of membranes of plants, animals, and other life forms. PS is also involved in moving signals through brain cells. It is isolated from soybeans and egg yolks.

Phosphatidylserine may be important for Alzheimer's prevention and treatment because it restores acetylcholine release in aging rats by maintaining an adequate supply of the molecule. Its presence also increases the availability of choline (one of the building blocks of the brain chemical acetylcholine) for new acetylcholine production. Rat experiments indicate that PS treatment prevents the age-related reduction in dendritic spine density (the branches of cells that interconnect with other cells) in the rat hippocampus. PS was found to restore metabolic activity in brain cells of aging rats.

Phosphatidylserine has demonstrated some usefulness in humans in treating cognitive impairment, including Alzheimer's disease, age-associated memory impairment and some non-Alzheimer's dementias. Several double-blind studies suggest that phosphatidylserine can help maintain cognitive function in older individuals and may be able to improve memory and learning skill in some. These results, while encouraging, have not been dramatic. In the largest multicenter study to date of phosphatidylserine and Alzheimer's disease, 142 subjects aged forty to eighty were given 200 mg of phosphatidylserine or a placebo each day over a three-month period. Those treated with phosphatidylserine exhibited improvement in several items on the scales normally used to assess Alzheimer's status. The differences between the placebo and experimental groups were small but statistically significant. Researchers directing a smaller study, also achieving statistical significance with respect to several measures, characterized the therapeutic effects of phosphatidylserine in their Alzheimer's subjects as "mild." Other studies examining PS have not been as rigorously executed.

Despite promising evidence, the FDA has not endorsed this compound as meeting rigorous scientific standards to merit approval as a treatment or prevention for Alzheimer's, citing flaws in the methods of study design and execution. A report issued by the FDA states, "Based on its evaluation of the totality of the publicly available scientific evidence, the agency concludes that there is not significant scientific agreement among qualified experts that a relationship exists between phosphatidylserine and reduced risk of dementia or cognitive dysfunction."

There are not presently any prevention trials of phosphatidylserine against Alzheimer's. To date, phosphatidylserine is considered relatively safe and has no major counterindications, making it a good candidate for further research in the context of Alzheimer's therapy and prevention. There are no reported drug, nutritional supplement, food, or herbal interactions with phosphatidylserine. A target dose would be 100 to 200mg.

Supplements That May Be Helpful from a Scientific Perspective but Are Still Unproven

Following are some of the "brain supplements" whose track records in dementia and cognitive health are not proven but that have some potential, given how they work biologically.

DHEA

Dehydroepiandrosterone (DHEA) and its metabolite, DHEA-S, together abbreviated DHEAS, are the most abundant steroids produced by the human adrenal glands and gonads (testicles in men, ovaries in women). Produced in the brain and termed *neuros-teroids,* their physiologic functions remain unclear. DHEAS is part of a group of steroid hormones that may be important with how bodies respond to stress, and have recently attracted widespread scientific and lay attention. This is because it is likely that stress and glucocorticoids may play an important role in memory and cognitive performance in neuropsychiatric conditions such as dementia, as well as in depression, post-traumatic stress disorder, and Cushing's disease (which involves the adrenal glands that sit on top of the kidneys). Also, circulating levels in the blood of DHEAS are highest when people are in their twenties and decrease progressively as men and women get older. By age sixty-five, when the incidence of Alzheimer's begins to rise, these hormones are down to 10 to 20 percent of their levels in young adults. Although it isn't a uniform finding, some studies have discovered that people with Alzheimer's tend to have especially low-serum DHEAS levels. This, in turn, led to the speculation that replacement dosing with supplemental DHEA might have beneficial therapeutic effects. However, as you read about these study findings, keep in mind that sex and age make big differences in hormone research. One group of investigators did not find a difference in DHEA serum concentrations between Alzheimer's patients and age-matched controls, but did find that the DHEA/stress-steroid cortisol was lower among Alzheimer's patients than in their non-demented peers, especially among women.

In 1998, a group of scientists demonstrated that elderly humans with prolonged cortisol (stress steroid) elevations showed reduced volume of the hippocampus (the seat of memory in the brain) and deficits in hippocampus-dependent memory tasks, compared with controls who had normal cortisol concentrations. The authors speculated that perhaps DHEA medication and its anti-steroid mechanisms might protect the hippocampus against elevated basal cortisol in patients with Alzheimer's, a theory reinforced by preclinical studies showing DHEAS to have brain protective effects. In laboratory studies, DHEAS has also been shown to enhance cellular function in the hippocampus, to protect against oxidative stress, to increase availability of the protective growth factors, and to decrease production and deposition of beta-amyloid protein.

Despite these bullish lab findings, DHEA studies in humans have had mixed results. Some clinical trials have suggested that DHEA treatment increases memory function, sense of well-being, energy, and mood in healthy elderly volunteers. Other studies have shown no benefit at all. Definitive answers regarding DHEA's cognitive and mood effects have remained elusive.

With these mixed findings in mind, a really good clinical trial was performed at the University of California–San Francisco. The researchers speculated that even if DHEAS levels were lower in patients suffering from Alzheimer's, then restoring hormone levels to those seen in younger, healthy people might still have beneficial effects in this disease. Designed to assess DHEA's efficacy and tolerability in patients with Alzheimer's, the study looked at whether DHEA treatment would improve cognitive function and the severity level of the Alzheimer's if tested alongside subjects receiving a placebo. Investigators enrolled fifty-eight Alzheimer's patients for six months and administered 100 mg daily of DHEA to roughly half, while the other half received a placebo. All underwent the same standard memory/cognitive tests done in clinical trials. Although DHEA was relatively well tolerated among the participants, investigators saw no appreciable clinical benefit on memory/cognitive tests or on mood ratings and concluded that DHEA was not an effective potential treatment for Alzheimer's.

Another four-week study of DHEA in both demented and non-demented elderly participants also yielded no cognitive or mood changes. The only evidence of dementia-improving properties comes from a very small sample size (seven individuals) in an open-label trial, and the mood and memory improvements noted were modest.

It seems that as with estrogen replacement therapy, there is as yet no compelling evidence for DHEA in treating individuals with Alzheimer's. With weak evidence of treatment benefit, it is hard to take the larger leap forward on DHEA as a preventative agent. Its use in prevention of Alzheimer's is speculative at this point. Therefore, 100 mg would be a reasonable dose.

Choline and Phosphatidylcholine (Lecithin)

As the body ages, according to the cholinergic theory of Alzheimer's disease, the brain produces less of the neurotransmitter acetylcholine. This depletion may precipitate eventual short- and long-term memory loss. Choline (delivered with the compounds phosphatidylcholine, aka lecithin) helps synthesize the neurotransmitter acetycholine in the brain and acts as a lipid transport in the liver. Phosphatidylcholine is important for normal cellular membrane composition and repair. Phosphatidylcholine is also the major delivery form of the essential nutrient choline. The body produces choline naturally, but it is also present in dietary sources such as egg yolks and soy products.

Because of choline and phosphatidylcholine's role in acetylcholine production and preservation, Alzheimer's researchers have been looking to these compounds for some therapeutic benefit for a long time. There is some anecdotal evidence that phosphatidylcholine may be useful in the management of Alzheimer's disease and some other cognitive disorders, but study after study has turned up little evidence that choline can improve cognitive health or reduce risk of dementia. Clinical trials have shown that it did not significantly improve cognition in the treatment of Alzheimer's. This may be attributed in part to the fact that choline administered from outside the brain does not cross into the brain.

That said, this compound is safe and nontoxic, and should always be taken with vitamin B_5, folate, and vitamin B_{12} for proper absorption. Choline and lecithin have been investigated in a variety of health conditions including liver disease, hepatitis, cancer, and degenerative diseases like Huntington's disease.

At present, there is no clinical evidence published demonstrating convincing evidence of choline or lecithin as a preventative agent against Alzheimer's. Despite limited objective evidence that choline and phosphatidylcholine can improve cognitive measures or treat/prevent this disease, it is by far and away the most common supplement promoted for cognitive/memory health and is the cornerstone of most memory-enhancing formulations. At the end of the day, this supplement has little risk of adverse or toxic effects but consumers should be mindful that the positive result may be minimal.

DMAE

Dimethylaminoethanol (DMAE) is related to choline and is a precursor to the neurotransmitter acetylcholine. It is found naturally in sardines and anchovies. DMAE is believed to be chemically altered in the body to produce choline in the brain. DMAE is processed by the liver into choline; however, because the choline molecule is charged, it cannot pass the blood-brain barrier into the brain. Evidence suggests that DMAE crosses the blood-brain barrier more effectively than choline does, enabling it to reach the brain and increase the brain's choline levels more efficiently.

Short-term studies show that patients taking DMAE show an increase in vigilance and alertness, as well as uplifting mood. Long-term studies, however, are more equivocal. Some animal studies showed that DMAE can increase one's life span. There are still no randomized controlled clinical trials for DMAE to be used for the treatment or prevention of Alzheimer's. With the uncertainty of whether this protective could be extrapolated to humans, DMAE supplementation is not generally recommended as a preventive strategy for Alzheimer's.

Grapeseed Extract and Quercetin

Grapeseed extract is the only plant-based antioxidant powerhouse and as such has been the subject of much positive attention as a therapy for atheroscleroris, certain cancers, eye conditions, and capillary disorders. Grapeseed extract is rich in chemicals known as polyphenols (including the subclass of plant flavonoids called proanthocyanidins, or PCOs), which are recognized to be effective antioxidants. This means that polyphenols protect body cells from damage caused by the chemical process called oxidation, which produces oxygen free radicals. Grapeseed has an antioxidant power 50 percent higher than that of vitamins C or E.

For example, human case reports and results from some laboratory and animal studies appear to show that grapeseed extract may help to prevent and treat heart diseases such as high blood pressure and high cholesterol. Antioxidants in grapeseed extract may help prevent changes, including damage to blood vessels, which may contribute to the development of heart disease. Substances in grapeseed extract may also block the effects of enzymes that process fats, including cholesterol, from the diet. Consequently, less fat may be absorbed and more may be eliminated from the body. Other research shows that grapeseed extract may help to prevent or control damage to body cells caused by drugs, pollution, tobacco, and other toxins.

Although grapeseed extract sounds appealing because of its potent antioxidant properties, research on it as dementia therapy is limited. There are no studies reported on grapeseed extract as a treatment or prevention of Alzheimer's. A recommended daily dosage for preventative antioxidant effect is 50 mg, and for therapeutic uses, between 150 and 300 mg.

I discussed quercetin briefly in chapter 12. Quercetin is a flavonoid, also derived from grapes, that forms the chemical root for many other flavonoids, including the citrus flavonoids rutin, hesperidin, naringin, and tangeritin. Quercetin is found to be the most active of the flavonoids in studies, and many plants owe their medicinal qualities to their high quercetin content. Quercetin has demonstrated significant anti-inflammatory activity because of direct inhibition of several initial processes of inflammation. Quercetin may also have positive effects in combating or helping to prevent cancer, inflamed prostate, heart disease, cataracts, allergies/inflammations, and respiratory diseases such as bronchitis and asthma. Foods rich in quercetin include apples, black and green teas, onions, raspberries, red wine, red grapes, citrus fruits, broccoli and other cruciferous/leafy green vegetables, and cherries.

Despite its potent antioxidant properties, data on quercetin as a treatment or preventative for Alzheimer's are sparse. There are no published studies on quercetin's effects upon this disease. A typical dose is 120 mg.

Acetyl-L-Carnitine (ALC)

ALC plays an important role in cellular energy production and regulation, and animal studies point to evidence that it can actually reverse some age-related brain cell damage. The acetyl component of acetyl-L-carnitine provides for the formation of the neurotransmitter acetylcholine. ALC is an important molecule in the parts of cells called *mitochondria*, the batteries inside every cell. When the mitochondria don't operate properly, cells do not function well because they don't have sufficient energy to conduct normal processes. The mechanism of action is not exactly known. Some have hypothesized that ALC improves the efficiency of CNS cells' mitochondrial/energy production. Others have said that it stabilizes brain cell membranes. Finally, ALC is said to decrease accumulations in cells of toxic fatty acids.

Although ALC may boost levels of the neurotransmitters acetylcholine and dopamine, among human subjects with probable age-related dementia, ALC therapy has been linked with only modest gains in memory tests. Several studies have now demonstrated some positive effects of acetyl-L-carnitine supplements in Alzheimer's patients, especially with regard to tasks involving attention and concentration. In a clinical trial of thirty patients with mild-to-moderate dementias or Alzheimer's disease, there were significant, positive results as measured by some of the neuropsychological tests used in the study. In another clinical trial of 130 patients with Alzheimer's disease, a slower rate of deterioration was observed in thirteen of fourteen measures studied at the end of its one-year study. In yet another clinical trial of acetyl-L-carnitine administered to seven probable Alzheimer's disease patients who were then compared to five placebo-treated probable Alzheimer's patients and twenty-one age-matched healthy controls over the course of one year, the acetyl-L-carnitine-treated patients showed significantly less deterioration in their memory and other cognitive test scores.

ALC was then developed and branded under the name ALCAR. Clinical trials of ALC as a potential treatment for Alzheimer's were then conducted. Evidence of ALCAR's efficacy is not very substantial or convincing. Moreover, some evidence suggests that it actually hastens the cognitive decline in some older-onset Alzheimer's patients (who compose the bulk of the population that contracts the disease). A one-year clinical trial showed that ALCAR (1 g three times a day) failed to decrease the rate of decline in early onset Alzheimer's patients. But a careful analysis of the data suggested some benefit in younger people suffering from Alzheimer's, and a follow-up study looking specifically at ALC in younger people suffering from Alzheimer's was done. In that trial, ALCAR had no clinically meaningful benefit, either.

In summary, ALC has potential beneficial effects as a treatment for Alzheimer's disease, but clinical evidence of benefit in humans is mixed with only modest benefits at best. No evidence is available that ALC prevents or delays Alzheimer's.

ALC is relatively well tolerated. Research into potential salutary effects of ALC supplements in healthy, nondemented adults is still needed. The target dose would be 3 g daily.

Vinpocetine

Vinpocetine is an alkaloid derived from a member of the periwinkle family (Vinca minor). Vinpocetine has several possible actions, including increasing cerebral blood flow and metabolism, and as an anticonvulsant, cognition enhancer, neuroprotector, and antioxidant. Vincamine, the parent compound of vinpocetine, is believed to be a cerebral *vasodilator* (meaning opener of blood vessels).

Several mechanisms have been proposed for the possible actions of vinpocetine. Vinpocetine works by increasing blood flow to the brain and promoting the brain's use of oxygen. It thins blood, dilates blood vessels, and protects neurons from toxic injury. It also has antioxidant effects. In some studies, vinpocetine has demonstrated antioxidant activity equivalent to that of vitamin E. It crosses into the brain and seems to be readily taken up by cerebral tissue.

Vinpocetine is prescribed in Europe and Mexico for cognitive and cerebrovascular conditions (that is, vascular dementia). In the United States, it is sold as a dietary supplement and promoted to address Alzheimer's disease, memory problems, stroke, and tinnitus (ringing in the ears). Several small studies, in both animals and humans, have reported significant vinpocetine-associated protective effects in ischemic stroke.

There is some evidence that vinpocetine may be useful in some other cerebral maladies. In one multicenter, double-blind, placebo-controlled study lasting sixteen weeks, 203 patients described as having mild to moderate "psychosyndromes" (not well defined in the study), including primary dementia, were treated with varying doses of vinpocetine or a placebo. Using "global improvement" scales and cognitive performance tests, researchers observed significant improvement in the vinpocetine-treated group. Three 10 mg doses daily were as effective as or more effective than were three 20 mg doses daily. Similarly impressive results were found in another clinical trial testing vinpocetine versus a placebo in elderly patients with cerebrovascular and central nervous system degenerative disorders. Despite claims to the contrary, studies to date have not produced evidence showing that vinpocetine is of benefit in Alzheimer's patients. No studies are reported investigating vinpocetine as a preventative agent against this disease.

Adverse reactions appear to be rare. They include nausea, dizziness, insomnia, drowsiness, dry mouth, and a temporary drop in blood pressure. Don't take vinpocetine if you're taking any type of blood-thinning medication (the drug may decrease platelet aggregation, inhibiting clot formation).

Since vinpocetine has come up short in studies with Alzheimer's disease, this compound should not be taken at this time with Alzheimer's prevention in mind, but a typical dose would be 30 mg a day.

Resveratrol

Resveratrol is a naturally occurring *phytoalexin* produced by some higher plants. Phytoalexins are chemical substances produced by plants as a defense against infection by microorganisms, such as fungi. Scientific studies have reported a number of beneficial health effects. Reservatol has been shown to have anticancer, antiviral, neuroprotective, antiaging, anti-inflammatory and life-prolonging effects. Epidemiological, in vitro, and animal studies suggest that a high resveratrol intake may contribute to a reduced incidence of cardiovascular disease, and a reduced risk for cancer.

Some of the beneficial effects of wine were discussed in chapter 12. Resveratrol is found in the skin of red grapes and, as a constituent of red wine, may explain the "French paradox" that the incidence of coronary heart disease is relatively low in southern France despite high dietary intake of saturated fats. The concentration of resveratrol in red wine is much higher than that of white wine. The main difference between red and white wine production, besides the grapes used, is that for red wine the skins and seeds are involved in the process, whereas white wine is mainly prepared from the juice, essentially avoiding the inclusion of grape skins and seeds. During the winemaking process, resveratrol, as well as other polyphenols that include quercetin, catechins, gallocatechins, procyanidins and prodelphidins (condensed tannins), are extracted from the grape skins via a process called *maceration*. Resveratrol is also found in peanuts, blueberries, some pines, such as Scots pine and eastern white pine, and the roots and stalks of giant knotweed and Japanese knotweed, called *hu zhang* in China.

Resveratrol has potent anticancer properties, demonstrating that it can inhibit the growth of several cancer cell lines and tumors, human leukemia cell lines and some breast carcinoma cells among them. More preliminary yet are findings that resveratrol may also stimulate the immune system. Resveratrol may also have protective effects against heart disease. Other studies, in animals and in vitro, have shown that resveratrol can inhibit the oxidation of LDL-cholesterol and, more recently, that it can reduce by 70 to 90 percent the thickening of the walls of the arteries believed to be one of the requisites of arterial blockage. The mechanisms of resveratrol's effect on life extension, at least in bacteria, worms, and fish, are not yet fully understood. Finally, resveratrol has recently been reported to be effective against neuronal cell dysfunction and cell death, and may be of use for diseases such as Huntington's and Alzheimer's.

Although resveratrol appears promising, at least theoretically, as a potential treatment or preventative for Alzheimer's, no clinical research data yet exists to help us make a determination as to its usefulness. Some of the anti-Alzheimer's properties were discussed in chapter 12. Clinical trials to investigate the benefits of resveratrol as a treatment for Alzheimer's are set to get under way. There is no current data available of resveratrol's ability to prevent Alzheimer's. Nevertheless, it is well tolerated. The typical dose would be 20 mg daily.

Should You Take These Supplements?

Think back to the table at the beginning of this chapter: remember how unbalanced it was? As things stand now, when it comes to Alzheimer's research, the scales are tipped in the direction of unproven or weakly supported supplements. That is unfortunate, as many of these substances may have theoretic benefit that is simply untested to date in a clinical study. Without compelling clinical data, however, it is difficult to recommend some supplements with an eye toward Alzheimer's prevention. In the future, science may be able to bring more weight to some of the claims made about the substances on the left-hand side. But for now, keep this chapter in mind as you make decisions about adding supplements to your daily dementia prevention regimen, and always discuss any over-the-counter supplement with your health-care provider or pharmacist before beginning to take it. Sometimes supplements can interact with prescription medications or can cause unpleasant side effects, and therefore should be taken only after careful review with a medical professional.

Final Thoughts and Recommendations

- Be discerning about claims made for dietary supplements. There is very little objective evidence that any supplements have been proven to prevent Alzheimer's.
- For omega-3 fatty acids, focus on taking supplements high in

DHA. Your target is at least 1,000 mg daily of DHA. Most omega-3 formulations have high amounts of EPA, so read the label.

- Consider taking 400 to 800 mg of curcumin daily.

- If you are not on blood-thinning medication, consider taking ginkgo biloba supplements, 120 mg daily.

- Huperzine A may actually help memory. The recommended daily dose is 200 to 400 mcg daily.

- Phosphatidylserine has been shown to have mild benefit in a few Alzheimer's studies. The target dose is 200 mg daily.

- Although it has not been proven to prevent Alzheimer's, resveratrol has attractive if not entirely proven anti-Alzheimer's properties. The target dose is 20 mg daily.

- DHEA has not shown as much promise as had been hoped for.

- Choline and lecithin (aka phosphatidylcholine), although safe and theoretically desirable, do not show strong evidence of benefit to cognitive outcomes in rigorously conducted clinical trials.

- More investigation is needed regarding grapeseed extract/quercetin, acetyl-I-carnitine, DMAE, and vinpocetine.

- Ask your doctor or pharmacist before taking any supplement.

PART IV

If You Have Alzheimer's Disease

19

Get Help: Alzheimer's Is Treatable

M any who face Alzheimer's do not know where to turn and who to seek help from. This chapter provides a step-by-step action plan to help you navigate this scary disease. The most important thing to realize is that Alzheimer's disease can be diagnosed reasonably accurately and it can be managed with treatments that can modestly improve your quality of life.

Know these facts:

- Alzheimer's disease can be diagnosed during life.
- Alzheimer's disease is a treatable disease.
- Medications are available to treat the disease, although family members should have modest expectations.
- Alzheimer's disease can have behavioral complications, which are also treatable.

It is time for us collectively to rethink Alzheimer's disease. One of the most important things to consider in this rethinking is that Alzheimer's is not treatable. It is. Here are some myths and facts about Alzheimer's treatments.

Treatment Myths and Facts

Myth: Alzheimer's cannot be treated.

Not true: There are now medications to treat Alzheimer's.

Myth: Treatment simply extends the duration of the illness.
Not necessarily true: Current treatment can modestly improve quality of life.

Myth: Alzheimer's is simply a diagnosis of exclusion.
Partially true: Historically, that is how we diagnosed Alzheimer's disease. But new technology and biomarkers are allowing us to pinpoint a diagnosis with greater accuracy.

Myth: Alzheimer's can only be diagnosed after death.
Partially true: While Alzheimer's disease can be definitely diagnosed at autopsy, that is not the only time it can be diagnosed— we can diagnose Alzheimer's disease nowadays during life with greater than 90 percent accuracy.

Myth: People don't die from Alzheimer's.
Not true: People die from Alzheimer's because it leads to loss of activities of daily living (dressing, bathing, toileting, grooming), then loss of mobility, then becoming bed bound. Ultimately, being bed bound leads to infections that can cause death, but the primary reason a person becomes bed bound is from the Alzheimer's.

Know the Signs and Symptoms of Alzheimer's

In the first chapter, I discussed the many signs and indicators of Alzheimer's and dementia you should watch for in yourself and loved ones. When you recognize that you or your loved one has memory loss, do not ignore it. Early diagnosis is important, so patients and families can seek appropriate evaluations and care as well as plan for the future. To get a feeling of whether you are headed toward Alzheimer's disease, here are two questionnaires that you can use on yourself or on a loved one to determine if symptoms of memory loss portend a more ominous condition. The first is partly derived from the Alzheimer's Association's Web site (www.alz.org).

Do You Have Alzheimer's Disease?

Memory loss that affects job skills:

- Have you been laid off or demoted, or do you find yourself moving from job to job because you cannot remember tasks?
- Do you have trouble learning new tasks that you would have learned easily before?

Difficulty performing familiar tasks:

- Have you given up or significantly reduced activities such as cooking, check writing and other finance-related tasks, supermarket shopping, and home maintenance?
- Are you struggling to do these tasks?
- Do family members have to supervise tasks such as cooking because of safety hazards?
- Are you having trouble completing tasks?
- Are family members concerned about your driving abilities? Have you been in minor motor vehicle accidents that would not typically have happened in the past?
- Are family members noticing that meals do not taste the same or that the housekeeping has slipped?

Problems with language:

- Are people completing your sentences?
- Are you losing your train of thought frequently?
- Are you using general references when talking about people (e.g., "that guy," rather than a name)?
- Do you struggle to find words and names on a daily basis?
- Are you having trouble naming familiar people such as your children or grandchildren?

Disorientation to time and place:

- Are you having trouble tracking days and dates?
- Do you get lost in familiar places?

- Do you have trouble tracking appointments?
- Are you looking at the calendar or newspaper daily or hourly to check the date? Do you confuse the days of the week, or dates, or the months of the year?
- Do you ask loved ones for the days and date?

Poor or decreased judgment:

- Are you forgetting to pay bills?
- Are you making ill-advised decisions about investments?
- Are you making inappropriate purchases?
- Are you entering every sweepstakes, when you had not done so in the past?
- Are you consenting to every telesolicitation?
- Are you giving more money to charities or others than you can afford?

Problems with abstract thinking:

- Are you having trouble grasping abstract thoughts?
- Do you have trouble comprehending complex items such as investments, nuances of storylines, or subtleties of inter-relationships?

Misplacing things:

- Do you spend a lot of time every day looking for keys or glasses?
- Do you misplace objects frequently (once a week or more)?
- Do others spend time frequently helping you look for objects?
- Do you place objects in places that are not typical, such as utensils in refrigerators or garments in kitchen cupboards?

Changes in mood or behavior:

- In addition to memory loss, do you suffer from depression and/or anxiety?
- Are you losing interest in activities?
- Are you less inclined to socialize with others?
- Are you becoming more withdrawn?
- Are you more anxious or nervous when separated from others?

Changes in personality:

- Frequently, families comment about increased irritability and hostility toward loved ones. This is a manifestation of a common cycle of events. Here is an example: (Patient) "Dear, when is my appointment?" (Spouse) "I have told you five times already. It is tomorrow morning!" (Patient) "No, you haven't! You are lying. I would remember if you told me. . . ." Do you find this kind of conversation taking place?

- Are you more impatient than you were before?
- Are you more suspicious of others?
- Are you becoming paranoid?
- Do you have false beliefs (theft, abandonment, infidelity)?

My colleagues and I at Sun Health Research Institute developed an alternative questionnaire. We call it the Alzheimer's Questionnaire (AQ). It is a series of yes or no questions. The yes answers are assigned points as indicated in the last column. It is intended to be administered to an informant (not the person with the memory loss). After you take the survey on behalf of someone you are concerned about, if the score is greater than 10 points, then you should have the person with the memory loss seek medical attention. If the score is less than 5, then there is low probability that the memory loss represents Alzheimer's disease.

Alzheimer's Questionnaire

	YES	NO	WEIGHTED SCORE
MEMORY			
Does the patient have memory loss?			1
If so, is his or her memory worse than a few years ago?			1
Does the patient repeat questions OR statements OR stories in the same day?			2
Have you had to take over keeping track of events OR appointments? OR Does the patient forget appointments?			1

(continued)

Alzheimer's Questionnaire *(continued)*

	Yes	No	Weighted Score
Does the patient misplace items more than once a month? OR Does the patient misplace objects so that he or she cannot find them?			1
Does the patient suspect others are moving, hiding, or stealing items when he or she cannot find them?			1

ORIENTATION

	Yes	No	Weighted Score
Does the patient frequently have trouble knowing the day, date, month, year, time? OR Does the patient have to use cues like a newspaper or a calendar to know the day and date more than once a day?			2
Does the patient become disoriented in unfamiliar places?			1
Does the patient become more confused outside the home or when traveling?			1

FUNCTIONAL ABILITY

	Yes	No	Weighted Score
Excluding physical limitations (for example, tremor, hemiparesis, etc.), does the patient have trouble handling money (tips, calculating change)?			1
Excluding physical limitations (for example, tremor, hemiparesis, etc.), does the patient have trouble paying bills or doing finances OR Are family members taking over finances because of concerns about ability?			2
Does the patient have trouble remembering to take medications or keeping track of medications taken?			1

Alzheimer's Questionnaire

	Yes	No	Weighted Score
Is the patient having difficulty driving? OR Are you concerned about the patient's driving? OR Has the patient stopped driving for reasons other than physical limitations?			1
Is the patient having trouble using appliances (for example, microwave, oven, stove, remote control, telephone, alarm clock)?			1
Excluding physical limitations, is the patient having difficulty completing home repair or other home-related tasks (for example, housekeeping)			1
Excluding physical limitations, has the patient given up or significantly reduced recreational activities such as golfing, dancing, exercising, or crafts?			1
VISUOSPATIAL			
Is the patient getting lost in familiar surroundings (own neighborhood)?			2
Does the patient have a decreased sense of direction?			1
LANGUAGE			
Does the patient have trouble finding words other than names?			1
Does the patient confuse names of family members or friends?			2
Does the patient have difficulty recognizing people familiar to him/her?			2

If, on the basis of these questionnaires, it is apparent that you or a loved one has symptoms of memory loss indicating potential Alzheimer's disease, then take the next questionnaire to assess what risk factors you or your loved one have for developing Alzheimer's disease.

Assess Your Risk of Getting Alzheimer's

RISK	YES	NO	SCORE
A mother, father, sister, or brother with Alzheimer's			3.0
A history of head injury with loss of consciousness			2.0
Age greater than 65			1.0
Age greater than 75			4.0
Age greater than 85			16.0
Education less than 7 years			3.6
Female gender			1.5
Systolic blood pressure greater than 140mmHg			2.2
BMI greater than 30kg/m2			2.3
Cholesterol >6.5 mmol/L			1.9
APO-Eε4 positive			2.4
History of stroke			4.0
History of heart attack			2.5
Untreated type 2 diabetes			3.0
Limited physical activity			1.7
Continuing to smoke			2.3
Total			

Partly derived from *Preventing Alzheimer's* by W. Rodman Shankle, Daniel Amen, and M. Kivepelto, et al. 2006. Risk score for the prediction of dementia risk in 20 years among middle aged people: a longitudinal, population based study. *Lancet Neurology* 5: 735–741.

Each yes is assigned a score number. Add them together. If your score is less than 5, then the risk is low. If your score is 5 to 12, then the risk is moderate. If your score is above 12, the risk is high.

See Your Doctor and Get Treatment

The first step is to see your primary care physician and ask for an evaluation, which is typically done by a neurologist, psychiatrist, or geriatrician.

If you are at all concerned that the evaluation by your doctor is lacking or there is uncertainty regarding the diagnosis or treatment, call the Alzheimer's Association national line (312) 335-8700 or the toll-free help line (800) 272-3900 to get the phone number of the local office nearest you. The local chapter keeps a list of physicians that specialize in evaluating and treating Alzheimer's.

The evaluation is more than simply asking your doctor whether you have memory problems. Physicians rely on a careful medical history, a physical examination, and certain laboratory tests to confirm the presence of disabling memory and thinking problems.

Besides an extensive history, a detailed physical and neurological examination is appropriate. This will include a simple bedside memory test; the most common one used is the Mini Mental State Examination (MMSE), but there are alternatives to this test.

You should also undergo a series of tests, including blood tests (as mentioned in chapter 4), plus brain scans such as CT, MRI, or even a PET scan. Typically, a physician orders a CT scan or an MRI, both of which provide detailed images of the brain, allowing him or her to identify causes of dementia besides Alzheimer's disease, including signs of strokes, tumors, and hydrocephalus (water on the brain).

A PET scan is a functional image, which means that instead of taking a picture of the brain, it scans the metabolic activity of the brain. With a PET scan, radioactive sugar is injected into the blood stream. Since the brain metabolizes sugar readily, this radioactive sugar is taken up to the brain tissue instantly, revealing areas of brain tissue that are less metabolically active because of cells' dying or not working properly. In Alzheimer's, a person has reduced metabolism in certain brain structures, specifically in the parietal and temporal lobes. PET scans are now approved by Medicare and can improve accuracy of diagnosis up to 93 percent.

The figures below show a PET scan of a normal brain (on the left) and a brain with Alzheimer's (on the right). In the normal brain, the bright red areas are metabolically active. The areas of blue in the Alzheimer's brain indicate where diminished metabolic activity has been revealed by a lesser uptake of the radioactive sugar.

The first figure shows a PET scan of a normal brain. All areas of the cortex (the outer rim) are brightly lit, meaning that they are metabolically active.

The second figure shows a PET scan of an Alzheimer's brain. There are areas of the cortex that are darker, meaning that they are not metabolically active. There is a characteristic pattern of change on PET scans that indicates Alzheimer's disease.

Sometimes, you might need a more extensive evaluation, which could include neuropsychological testing or even a spinal tap. Such neuropsychological tests involve paper-and-pencil tests and usually last several hours. They are essentially mental probes of the brain to find out where deficiencies lie, and can distinguish dementia from depression and some types of dementia from one another, as well as gauge the severity of symptoms. Neuropsychological tests are particularly useful when there is a mixture of conditions (such as alcoholism mixed with Alzheimer's), and can be more sensitive than simple bedside tests that physicians perform in the office.

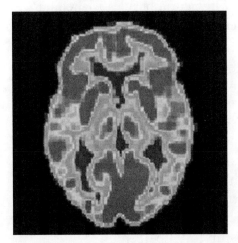

PET scan of a normal brain.

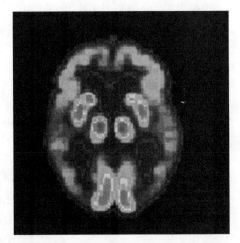

PET scan of an Alzheimer's brain.

Neuropsychological tests are performed by licensed practitioners called neuropsychologists, who perform the interview, conduct the tests (between two and eight hours in duration), and then generate a report for the patient's primary care physician.

Spinal fluid can also be used to diagnose Alzheimer's. A spinal tap (called *lumbar puncture* in medical parlance) is a procedure whereby spinal fluid is taken from the lower back. Spinal taps have been stigmatized by clumsy application in the past, but current methods make this a relatively safe procedure that can be done in a medical office and takes about fifteen to twenty minutes. Doctors can then analyze this spinal fluid and measure the changes in amyloid, tau, and phosphorylated tau that occur in Alzheimer's disease. Using the spinal fluid test, we can diagnose Alzheimer's with 88 to 90 percent accuracy, although the test is less accurate in discriminating one dementia type from another (only around 70 percent). For more information, ask your doctor or go to the Athena Diagnostics Web site (www.athenadiagnostics.com) and peruse the ADmark Alzheimer's Evaluation.

How accurate is an Alzheimer's diagnosis? Is it really only diagnosable at autopsy? As I mentioned in the myths and facts section earlier, Alzheimer's has been historically divided into probable, possible, and definite designations. The definite designation is assigned to autopsy or biopsy confirmation, leading to the popular belief that it cannot be diagnosed during life.

But using current technology, including imaging, neuropsychological testing, genotyping, and spinal fluid analysis, the accuracy of a life diagnosis of Alzheimer's can approach between 93 and 97 percent. So despite popular belief, Alzheimer's can be diagnosed fairly accurately.

Take Medications and Treatments

Goals for the treatment of Alzheimer's disease include improved memory, improved behavioral symptoms, preserving function (meaning present abilities), and slowed progression/decline.

The overall goal of treatment is not to add more years of life but to add better years. The life expectancy of a person with

Alzheimer's is roughly half as much as it would be without Alzheimer's. Thus, for example, a sixty-five-year-old without cancer has a twenty-year life expectancy; but with Alzheimer's, it would be ten years. Overall, treatment goals are focused on improving quality of life and making the years you do have left . . . much better!

The medications currently available have a modest but definite effect on Alzheimer's. They can improve such qualities as alertness, concentration, memory, and recall. It is uncommon for patients to get dramatically better, but it is common for patients to get somewhat better.

Nevertheless, it is important to adjust expectations. These drugs are not cure-alls. Consider these points when pursuing treatment. Taking Alzheimer's medication:

- Is not a panacea
- Is now a standard of care
- Should be started early and continued
- Should be used with lower expectations
- May delay nursing home placement
- Can be used to treat behavioral complications

The goals for treatment also depend on the stage of disease. For mild symptoms/early stages, the primary goal is to preserve whatever possible mental functions. For instance, if a person has stopped driving but is able to do other things, such as handle his or her finances, the goal of treatment is not to regain the driving ability, but rather to not lose ability to do finances. Studies of donepezil have revealed a delay in functional decline. For moderate-stage disease, your goal is to avoid the "Big Three." These are falls, incontinence, and behavioral disturbances. The big three are the principal reasons why people with Alzheimer's are placed into long-term care. By avoiding these three, the people stay happy and they tend to stay home longer.

At the time this book went to press, five medications had been approved for the treatment of Alzheimer's disease (the commercial brands follow the generic term in parentheses).

- Donepezil (Aricept)
- Rivastigmine (Exelon)
- Galantamine (Razadyne, formerly known as Reminyl)
- Tacrine (Cognex—rarely used anymore because of severe side effects)
- Memantine (Namenda)

Aricept, Exelon, Razadyne, and Cognex slow the breakdown of acetylcholine, the neurochemical in the brain that is responsible for memory. By preventing the breakdown of acetylcholine, these medications promote communication between cells. They are called *cholineterase inhibitors*. All are approved for mild to moderate Alzheimer's. Aricept is also approved for moderate to severe Alzheimer's. Cholinesterase inhibitors have been used as a treatment for Alzheimer's for almost fifteen years, which means that hundreds of thousands of people have taken these drugs at one time or another. These drugs do not stop Alzheimer's but they may slow it down.

This graph below summarizes the rate of decline of people with Alzheimer's. People taking the medications Aricept, Exelon, Razadyne, or Cognex decline at a slower rate than people without treatment.

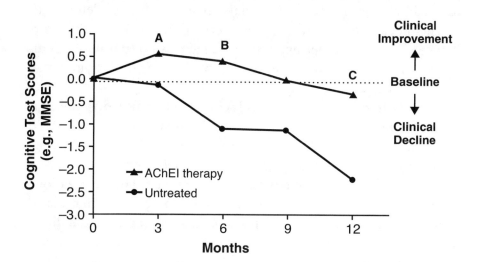

The upper line in the graph represents the people taking the medications and the lower line represents those taking the placebo. The upper line represents the group taking Aricept, Exelon, Razadyne, and Cognex all together. The graph illustrates that cholinergic medication actually slows the decline, although the disease is still progressing. This does not mean that the medicine is not working; it simply means that the disease is advancing despite the medications. Even though these drugs address just one aspect of the disease, they are an important option.

Namenda (memantine) is the newest medication, and works by a different mechanism than Aricept, Exelon, and Razadyne do. Namenda is currently approved for the treatment of moderate to severe Alzheimer's disease. Namenda is an *NMDA receptor antagonist*, which means that it protects brain cells from becoming overexcited (excitotoxicity). This overexcitement is related to the excess production of a brain chemical called glutamate. When there is an excess of glutamate, the brain cells take in too much calcium, causing them to die.

Behavioral Disturbances

One of the most common and distressing features of Alzheimer's is the development of behavioral disturbances. In fact, behavioral disturbances are one of the main reasons that patients with Alzheimer's are placed into long-term care. Behavioral disturbances include wandering, agitation, aggression, paranoia, delusions, anxiety, and hallucinations. People become restless, and may shadow or pace.

Treatment of these conditions is complex because most medications are not approved to treat behavioral symptoms, so instead we physicians can choose to treat the different components. Antidepressants are available to treat anxiety and agitation, and antipsychotic agents, such as risperidone (Risperdal), ziprazadone (Geodon), olanzapine (Zyprexa), quetiapine (Seroquel), and aripiprazole (Abilify) can be prescribed to treat paranoia, hallucinations, and delusions. These medications have side effects and complications, and need to be carefully monitored by your doctor. Medications to treat epilepsy, such as divalproex sodium (Depakote), can also be used in Alzheimer's patients to treat general agitation. For acute agitation (yelling, kicking, screaming), I prefer to give people a Valium-type sedative called lorazepam (Ativan) since it works quickly and is short acting.

For sleep disturbances that sometimes accompany Alzheimer's, you have to be careful. Melatonin has not been shown to be effective in treating sleep disturbances in Alzheimer's. And it is imperative that you avoid over-the-counter sleeping medications (such as anything with PM in its brand name), because all of them contain diphenhydramine (Benadryl), which blocks the effects of some of the Alzheimer's drugs and can make people worse. Try trazadone instead, or the newer romelteron (Rozerem).

You Are Not Alone

There are 4.5 million people with Alzheimer's, but that figure doesn't account for the millions of loved ones in their lives, the families and caretakers who are deeply affected by an Alzheimer's diagnosis. Alzheimer's is frightening. Although a lot of services are available, knowing where to turn can be bewildering. Below, I offer some places to start.

Web-based resources include:

- The Sun Health Research Institute: www.shri.org
- The Arizona Alzheimer's Disease Consortium: www.azalz.org
- The Alzheimer's Association: www.alz.org
- The Alzheimer's Disease Education and Referral Center (ADEAR); a service of the National Institute on Aging: www.alzheimers.org
- The Leeza Gibbons Memory Foundation: www.leezasplace .org
- The Alzheimer's Research Forum: www.alzforum.org
- Info regarding Aricept: www.aricept.com
- The National Institute of Aging Information Center: www.nia .nih.gov

- Other helpful publications are at: www.niapublications.org.
- Info regarding Exelon (Novartis) is at AlzheimersDisease .com: www.AlzheimersDisease.com.
- Alzheimer's Foundation of America: www.alzfdn.org
- National Family Caregivers Association: www.nfacares.org
- American Health Assistance Foundation: www.ahaf.org
- Info regarding Namenda (Forest Pharmaceuticals) is at: www .Namenda.com.
- Info regarding Razadyne/Reminyl (Ortho McNeil Neuro-logics): www.sharingcare.com
- AlzheimerSupport.com: www.alzheimersupport.com
- HealingWell.com: www.healingwell.com/alzheimers
- Topics.net: www.topix.net/health/alzheimers-disease
- The Alzheimer's Association Desert Southwest Chapter (Arizona and Southern Nevada): www.alzdsw.org
- The American Academy of Neurology: www.aan.com
- My Web site: www.the alzheimersanswer.com

Make Plans

When your diagnosis is made, you will need to have frank and often uncomfortable discussions with your family to plan your future care. In my practice, I recommend that families discuss: care options, driving, safety precautions, financial planning, and residential care options.

If you have been recently diagnosed with Alzheimer's, one of the first steps you must take is to make an appointment with an attorney. Elder-care attorneys are very experienced in planning for the future, and can advise on matters including durable and health-care powers of attorney (the latter of which is also known as a health-care proxy), guardianship, and the establishment of wills and trusts. Drawing up a living will and assigning a health-care power of attorney early will help to establish a chain of command if things get sour or troublesome. These decisions need to be made early because when serious complications occur (and they do), it is often difficult for both the patient and his or her family to think clearly. That is not the best time to be making health-care and long-term decisions. It is best to make them as soon as you can.

There is a fine and delicate line between being supervised by your family and having your own personal independence taken away from you for your own welfare. No single issue is more contentious than driving. This issue must be discussed early with your doctor and your family. Every state has different laws governing elder-related driving regulations and testing. To find out the laws in your state, check with the Department of Motor Vehicles. However, it is equally important for you to establish your own criteria for monitoring your ability to drive and coming to grips with the idea of surrendering your license. For more guidance, go to the American Academy of Neurology Web site, www.aan.com.

Do Not Give Up Hope

Although Alzheimer's is a frightening and life-changing disease for those who develop it and those who take care of them, there is hope. As I've shown in this book, what we know about the disease is growing faster than ever before, even as hundreds of thousands more physicians, researchers, long-term caregivers, and patient advocates join in discovering and developing paths to better treatment and prevention.

Final Thoughts and Recommendations

- Know the signs and symptoms of Alzheimer's, and do not ignore them.
- Alzheimer's disease is treatable. Prescription medications are available that improve the symptoms of the disease.
- Behavioral issues can overwhelm the caregivers, and need to be addressed immediately. Learn to recognize them early so you can head them off.
- Driving is by far and away the most contentious issue to

deal with in early Alzheimer's. Each state has different statutes and laws addressing driving and dementia. Discuss this issue early with your doctor.

- Plan for the future now. Take steps to deal with durable and health-care powers of attorney, as well as other fiduciary matters. Have a plan in place for health care and family emergencies.

- You are not alone. There is a plethora of services available— so do not be shy or proud about seeking help.

20

The Future of Alzheimer's Disease

When I first sat down to write this book, I had in mind both the person who, like me, has been the caretaker for someone with Alzheimer's disease and also the person who, like me, finds himself or herself middle-aged in a time of rapid and often confusing medical advances. Old age can seem both a very close reality and an ever-receding destination. As I began to write, I understood that the scope of this book is far larger. Along with my fellow dementia doctors, I have undertaken a global challenge, one that will affect all future generations and one that requires us to shift away from the way we providers and consumers of health care think about cures vs. prevention, terminal vs. chronic disease, and the economics of health and health care.

The unique and fundamental problem of health care is no longer just between ourselves and a general practitioner. There are decisions that will be made by governments, proposals drawn up by research scientists, protocols established by medical insurance groups, and research avenues pursued by pharmaceutical companies. These will intimately affect the very personal and daily act of living in good health or with disease. As we age, the following questions are likely to affect us all, whether or not we develop Alzheimer's: How many pill bottles will be by your bedside? How frequently will you have to go to the hospital because of illness? What will your co-payments and deductibles amount to? Should you draw up a living will? When will you prepare that guest bedroom for a home health care attendant or an aging parent? These are just examples of the many choices that we will have to make. And so it seems fitting that we should return, when closing this book, to talking about the chapters that have not yet been written—the future of Alzheimer's disease.

The Changing of the Guard: From a Terminal to a Chronic Disease

In our lifetime, Alzheimer's will come to be seen not as a terminal disease (such as Lou Gehrig's disease and certain types of cancer) but a chronic one (like diabetes or hypertension). Indeed, the day will come when Alzheimer's patients will go to the doctor for their annual checkup, get their refills at the pharmacy, and go on their way. "Chronic" means we will be able to manage it, monitor it, and stabilize it. Rather than seeking a single, one-size-fits-all cure for Alzheimer's, looking at the future of Alzheimer's in this way— from terminal to chronic—allows us to prepare our health-care infrastructure, health insurance paradigm, and caretaking system. Only then will we be ready for the large influx of chronic Alzheimer's patients who will live with and in relation to the disease, rather than in fear of it.

An analogous situation is leukemia. Leukemias are blood-borne cancers, and were uniformly fatal in the past. Nowadays, many types of leukemia are chronic and can be kept in remission with medication. Another example is HIV/AIDS. In the recent past, HIV/AIDS was a death sentence. With the advent of protease inhibitors and antiretroviral antibiotics, HIV/AIDS has been transformed into a chronic disease. That day is coming for Alzheimer's, and it is sooner than most people think.

The Next Wave of Treatment: Disease-Modifying Drugs

There are two models for tracking disease change over time in Alzheimer's. The first model is symptomatic. Here, a medication is administered to patients and their symptoms will show improvement over a period of time, but the rate of decline will be unaffected. Ultimately, the downward trajectory will run parallel to the untreated condition. The current medications used to treat Alzheimer's are largely considered symptomatic. That means that they improve symptoms for a period of time but may not change the trajectory (rate of decline). Not all of us agree with that standpoint, but that is how the drugs are marketed.

In contrast, disease-modifying medications are intended to affect the trajectory of decline such that over time, Alzheimer's patients on these medications continuously show a lesser rate of decline and a progressively greater preservation of cognition and function, compared with the health of untreated patients.

Clinical drug development is far enough along that we expect to see the first of the disease-modifying drugs approved by the FDA and put on the market by the end of this decade! This stems directly from our growing understanding of the complex biology of Alzheimer's disease. There are four drugs nearing approval. They include R-flurbiprofen (Flurizan), tramiprosate (Alzhemed), leuprolide, and statins. Flurizan, developed by Myriad Pharmaceuticals, is derived from an anti-inflammatory (NSAID—see chapter 16). Although it does not retain the anti-inflammatory properties (meaning it will not reduce the aches and pains of arthritis), it does modify the behavior of one enzyme critical to the production of the toxic amyloid that accumulates in Alzheimer's. Alzhemed, developed by Neurochem, works by blocking a protein called glycosaminoglycan (GAG) that facilitates amyloid clumping together to make plaque. This drug may prevent the amyloid from sticking together. Leuprolide, commonly used to treat prostate cancer in men and endometriosis in women, has been patented and licensed by a company called Voyager Pharmaceuticals as a treatment for Alzheimer's. Leuprolide works by preventing brain cells distressed by the amyloid from accumulating. It helps the brain cells get back to cell division and reproduction. This, in turn, might prevent the cells from dying. The last of the first wave of drugs likely to make it to the market include the statins (for example, Lipitor). I discussed the role of statins in detail in chapter 13.

The next wave behind those four drugs includes vaccine-based therapies, secretase inhibitors, immunological therapies, and biotech drugs in development. The vaccine-based therapies have been in development since the discovery of the concept in 1999. Scientists at Elan found that injecting amyloid into genetically engineered mice, as if it were an infection, resulted in the mice's bodies treating it as such and their immune systems revving up to clear the amyloid from the brain.

At that time, many of us were convinced we were on the verge of a cure. What followed was the development of a first-generation Alzheimer's vaccine. This vaccine entered into clinical trials in the fall of 2001 and nearly four hundred individuals were enrolled in a matter of weeks. While optimism was riding high, tragic news followed in its wake. In the spring of 2002, eighteen cases of encephalitis (a brain swelling and inflammation) were reported. The study was stopped immediately. Five of the encephalitis-affected participants died. However, when the autopsies were performed, there was clear and unmistakable evidence that the vaccine had worked. The plaques were gone! Other changes were unmistakable. For the other participants who received the vaccine and did not have these complications, their Alzheimer's actually stabilized. Overall, this first attempt, while devastating, propelled scientists to narrow their focus. That is where we are now. Scientists are now looking at passive immunization (infusion of the antibodies into the bloodstream) as a possible means to immunize against Alzheimer's. This is akin to certain types of treatments for rheumatoid arthritis and rare neurological conditions. It may provide a safer and more effective therapy to reverse the Alzheimer's cascade.

Other drugs are in the pipeline, which interrupt the primary biology of the disease; these are drugs that are able to arrest amyloid production in its early stages. That is what the secretase inhibitors do. Overall, there are more than thirty drugs in development and many hold real promise for the future.

For a disease as complex as Alzheimer's, no one pill will be a panacea. A disease this complex is likely to require a similarly complex treatment regimen, and future Alzheimer's treatment will probably resemble chemotherapy: a cocktail of medications, vitamins, supplements, and activities taken in very specific doses on an ongoing basis. The good news is that we may be really able to slow the disease, so that years of a life worth living will be reaped. The bad news is that the cost of treatment will escalate. Current treatment conservatively runs $250 per month without Medicare D. Costs will likely break at $600 to $800 per month or higher if all medications in the works are required to treat the disease. As yet, we have not even proven that this cocktail is safe.

Identifying Risk: Predicting Alzheimer's with Imaging and Biomarkers

In the first part of this book, I talked a lot about assessing your Alzheimer's risk. And in chapter 19, I offer a way for you to score how much risk you might have of developing Alzheimer's.

Identifying those at risk for Alzheimer's early and more accurately than we can now is a top priority of the medical community. Researchers are investigating the comparative predictive value of Alzheimer's tests on a series of fronts: biochemical tests, such as blood and cerebrospinal fluid, paper-and-pencil memory tests (neuropsychological tests), genetic testing, and neuroimaging, specifically electroencephalographs (EEG), MRIs, and PET scans.

What all these tests are looking for is a *biomarker* of Alzheimer's disease. According to the criteria set forth by the Alzheimer's Disease Neuroimaging Initiative (a multimillion dollar project put forth by the NIH and the pharmaceutical companies), an ideal biomarker is characterized by the following:

- It should detect a fundamental feature of the pathology that is activated in the course of Alzheimer's.

- It should be validated consistently in autopsy confirmed cases of the disease.

- It should be precise, able to distinguish Alzheimer's from other dementias and normal aging.

- It should be able to be detected at the disease stage where a proposed drug could have its maximum effect.

The APO-Eε4 allele, which I discussed earlier, is the best example of a biomarker for Alzheimer's. But how and when such genetic testing for Alzheimer's should be offered is a complex and ethically charged question without a clear answer. Current guidelines by major medical groups do not endorse testing for asymptomatic individuals. What can you or your doctor do with the information once it had been obtained? Can these early diagnoses, purely on the basis of a genetic profile, open the door to discrimination? This is an area of an ongoing debate in legal and philosophical circles.

Memory tests are more accurate and more predictive than ever before. In one study of the predictive validity of memory tests, a research group from the Sunnybrook and Women's College in Toronto looked at individual components of the diagnostic workup used in the Canadian Study of Health and Aging. In another, researchers applied correspondence analysis to the basic word memory test used by the National Institute of Aging. They detected mild cognitive impairment and found that these analyses boosted the accuracy rate of distinguishing between MCI and normal function to 97 percent, and between MCI and mild dementia to 98 percent.

Right now, the likelihood of finding a blood-based biomarker at present is unclear. The potential of such a biomarker is tantalizing. By measuring levels of toxic beta-amyloid protein in the blood, such a test could help shift Alzheimer's diagnosis from "terminal" to "chronic" by offering physicians and their patients an early, unambiguous, and noninvasive measure to assess their Alzheimer's risk. Although recent tests have shown inconclusive links between beta-amyloid protein plasma levels and likelihood of Alzheimer's development, these levels are so fundamental to Alzheimer's pathology that researchers are still looking at them.

At Mayo Clinic in Rochester, researchers have enrolled 1,600 people with normal cognitive function and 400 with mild cognitive impairment for a longitudinal study aimed at deducing an Alzheimer's risk equation. And in collaboration with Mayo's

Jacksonville site, researchers are enrolling participants for a study that will look at the validity of a predictive biomarker test.

As predictive tools, imaging technologies have shown more promise. The PET scan has been used for more than twenty years to study dementia by measuring glucose metabolic rates in different areas in the brain. In Alzheimer's, the temporal and parietal lobes, as well as the posterior cingulate cortex, show a slowdown in glucose processing, indicating less metabolic activity (this is bad), as illustrated in chapter 19.

This type of PET scan may be replaced in the near future by a PET scan called PIB-PET. PIB is an abbreviation for Pittsburgh Compound B (because it was invented at the University of Pittsburgh). PIB binds to amyloid, causing a PIB-PET to illuminate the amyloid in the brain. This is beautifully shown in the figure below.

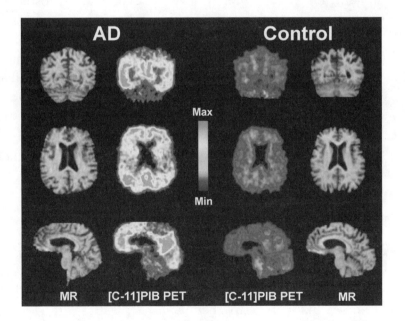

PIB-PET. This type of scan might be the future diagnostic test, as it actually identifies the amyloid plaques accumulating in the brain. On the left panel, the subject with Alzheimer's has a lot of bright (light areas) in the brain where the amyloid is. On the right panel, the normal elderly subject has a brain that is dark because there is no amyloid accumulating.

The bright areas on the left are areas where amyloid is being identified. The dark blue areas on the right are areas of brain that do not have amyloid. In this case, the brain on the left has Alzheimer's and the brain on the right is normal.

This technology will revolutionize how we diagnose Alzheimer's because it will permit us to precisely identify the changes occurring in the brains of Alzheimer's patients and diagnose the disease accurately, so treatment can start sooner.

Researchers are trying to fill those gaps by looking at the diagnostic value of imaging across large cohorts in longitudinal studies. The Alzheimer's disease Neuroimaging Initiative is an eight-hundred-person study conducted at sixty centers in North America that aims to measure the predictive value of MR and PET imaging, as well as other clinical markers, by studying a group of cognitively normal and MCI people over time.

As imaging techniques improve, we can expect such prospective longitudinal studies to shed more light on Alzheimer's progression early on. Imaging has already shown much promise as a predictive tool. My colleague Dr. Eric Reiman, of the Banner Alzheimer's Institute, performed PET scans on nondemented normal individuals who are carriers of the APO-Eε4 gene in their thirties, forties, and fifties. His team demonstrated that brain changes are detectable on PET scans years before symptoms would even manifest themselves. And, using the PIB-PET scan, researchers from the University of Pittsburgh and Washington University discovered the early signs of Alzheimer's in subjects without any cognitive symptoms. By comparing the amyloid burdens in the different brains, these scans matched up with diagnoses of MCI and Alzheimer's and helped researchers accurately predict conversion to MCI and Alzheimer's over time. These are just some of the ways that progress in neuroimaging is moving us closer to being able to predict who is likely to get Alzheimer's.

One day, you won't need a neurologist—all you will need is a PET scan.

At-Risk Profiling: The Upside and Downside

In the future, we will also train our sights on identifying at-risk individuals years or even decades before symptoms first appear. In time, we may even be able to estimate someone's lifetime risk of developing Alzheimer's. The upside here is that a person, knowing his or her risk of Alzheimer's, could benefit from the prevention recommendations in this book and implement them in hopes of delaying or preventing Alzheimer's altogether.

The major downside to at-risk profiling is the potential for discrimination. Imaging, like the other diagnostic tools I've discussed, comes with a hefty set of ethical questions. While the medical community was energized in 1993 with the discovery of the APO-Eɛ4 allele and is energized still by the prospect of saving lives by finding predictive tests for Alzheimer's, we must move forward with caution and awareness of the ethical quagmire that could form from invasive, incomplete, or ill-designed disease profiling.

Studies have shown that between one-quarter and one-half of cognitively normal individuals show Alzheimer's pathology at autopsy. And while this fact, along with the rapidly aging population, brings home the potential value of finding a predictive biomarker for the disease that could allow early intervention, a diagnosis of presymptomatic Alzheimer's is an ethically thorny goal. After all, we don't yet have a safe and effective treatment, and one may still be years away. So if we can tell an asymptomatic forty-year-old that he is at high-risk for developing Alzheimer's disease, but we cannot yet offer him a reliable, proven, safe, and effective treatment plan, what service have we done him? Medical records, employer-based health care, long-term care insurance, and privacy concerns further muddy this issue. What genetic counseling do we give him? Should he forgo having children out of his fear that he will pass along the Alzheimer's gene?

Science is racing forward, and we must allow time for the ethical and legal discussions around these issues to play catch-up. So for the moment, we in the Alzheimer's community move toward the blanket (that is, nonprofiled) approach to Alzheimer's prevention; better to do all things than only a few or nothing at all.

Prevention: A Continuing Challenge

In these last chapters, I discussed the Alzheimer's therapies available on the market today, and others at various stages of laboratory development, clinical trials, and approval that are coming down the pike.

But from both a timeline and an economic standpoint, the development of disease-modifying drug therapies is still costly. If one becomes available, the questions about presymptomatic testing and biomarkers I touched on earlier take on different weight. When should someone get tested? Will insurance companies cover preclinical treatment, and who will be able to afford it?

And so I return to the promise of prevention. From every angle, the work of delaying Alzheimer's symptoms through lifestyle, diet, environment, and health maintenance, even if biomarkers become available, remains the most financially and medically sound avenue for now. Doing so will buy us time to fill in the gaps in what we know about Alzheimer's pathology, such as how transgenic mice models differ from humans in dementia treatment. It will allow us time to improve available and new treatment methods.

And this will be no small task. Funding for large-scale clinical prevention trials is hard to obtain; after all, the very idea of prevention means that a profit-making prescription drug won't be needed in the end. Increased concerns about health profiling and lack of a disease-altering therapy makes recruitment for the large studies needed for future research a challenge, too. And finally, there is ultimate public-health paradox. It is hard to establish when prevention therapies are working. The fact that we don't get Alzheimer's doesn't mean that we know exactly why we didn't get it. Determining the neuroprotective powers of this or that therapy or environmental factor in patients without any symptoms is a Herculean task but a necessary goal toward managing and perhaps someday stamping out this disease.

Alzheimer's is a tragic disease that robs individuals of their lives, dignity, and memory and afflicts the loved ones that care for those with Alzheimer's. The promise of a future without terrible disease includes the possibility of prevention. Here, I have summarized the current thinking about prevention and provided recommendations in the hope that many, if not all of us, will live to see a world without Alzheimer's.

References

References are arranged by chapter and in approximate order of usage within each chapter.

1. Alzheimer's Disease

American Psychiatric Association. 1994. *American Psychiatric Association diagnostic and statistical manual of mental disorders.* 4th ed. Washington, DC: American Psychiatric Association.

Rabins, P. V., C. G. Lyketsos, and C. D. Steele. 2006. *Practical dementia care.* 2nd ed. New York: Oxford University Press.

American Medical Association. May 2004. *AMA dementia guide: Guide to diagnosis, management and treatment of dementia.* American Medical Association.

McKhann, G., D. Drachman, M. Folstein, et al. 1984. Clinical diagnosis of Alzheimer's disease report of the NINCDS-ADRDA Work Group under the auspices of the Department of Health and Human Services Task Force on Alzheimer's Disease. *Neurology* 34:939–44.

Salmon, D., R. Thomas, M. Pay, et al. 2002. Alzheimer's disease can be accurately diagnosed in very mildly impaired individuals. *Neurology* 59:1022–28.

Reisberg, B., J. Weigel, E. Franssen, et al. 2006. Clinical features of severe dementia-staging. In *Severe Dementia,* ed. A. Burns and B. Winblad, 95–127. Hoboken, NJ: John Wiley & Sons.

Auer, S. R., S. G. Sclan, R. A. Yaffee, and B. Reisberg. 1994. The neglected half of Alzheimer disease: cognitive and functional concomitants of severe dementia. *J Am Geriatr Soc* 42:1266–72.

Reisberg, B., E. Franssen, M. A. Shah, et. al. 2000. Clinical/STET diagnosis of dementia: A review. In *Dementia,* ed. M. Maj and N. Sartorius, 69–115. Hoboken, NJ: John Wiley & Sons,

Franssen, E. H., A. Kluger, C. L. Torossian, and B. Reisberg. 1993. The neurologic syndrome of severe Alzheimer's disease: Relationship to functional decline. *Arch Neurol* 50:1029–39.

Reisberg, B., S. Ferris, M. De Leon, and T. Crook. 1982. The global deterioration scale for assessment of primary degenerative dementia. *Am J Psychiatry* 139:1136–39.

——. 1988. Global deterioration scale (GDS). *Psychopharmacology Bulletin* 24:661–63.

Reisberg, B. 1988. Functional assessment staging (FAST). *Psychopharmacology Bulletin* 24:653–59.

Types of Dementia

Kalaria, R. N., and C. Ballard. 1999. Overlap between pathology of Alzheimer disease and vascular dementia. *Alzheimer Dis Assoc Disord* 13 Suppl 3:S115–23.

Roman, G. C., T. K. Tatemichi, T. Erkinjuntti, et al. 1993. Vascular dementia: Diagnostic criteria for research studies; Report of the NINDS-AIREN International Workshop. *Neurology* 43:250–60.

Erkinjuntti, T. 1993. Clinical criteria for vascular dementia: The NINDS-AIREN criteria, *Dementia* 5:189–92.

Lopez, O. L., M. R. Larumbe, J. T. Becker, et al. 1994. Reliability of NINDS-AIREN clinical criteria for the diagnosis of vascular dementia. *Neurology* 44:1240–45.

Ringholz, G. M. 2000. Diagnosis and treatment of vascular dementia. *Top Stroke Rehabil* 7:38–46.

McKhann, G. M., M. S. Albert, M. Grossman, B. Miller, D. Dickson, and J. Q. Trojanowski. 2001. Clinical and pathological diagnosis of frontotemporal dementia: report of the Work Group on Frontotemporal Dementia and Pick's Disease. *Arch Neurol* 58:1803–9.

Pfefer, A., E. Luczywek, M. Gotbiowski, K. Czyewski, and M. Barcikowska. 1999. Frontotemporal dementia: An attempt at clinical characteristics. *Dementia and Geriatric Cognitive Disorders* 10:217–20.

Brun, A., B. Englund, L. Gustafson, et al. 1994. Consensus statement: Clinical and neuropathological criteria for frontotemporal dementia; The Lund and Manchester groups. *J Neurol Neurosurg Psychiatr* 57:416–18.

Brun, A. 1993. Frontal lobe degeneration of the non-Alzheimer type, revisited. *Dementia* 4:126–31.

McKeith, I. G., D. Galasko , K. Kosaka, et al. 1996. Consensus guidelines for the clinical and pathologic diagnosis of dementia with Lewy bodies (DLB): Report of the consortium on DLB international workshop. *Neurology* 47:1113–24.

Aarsland, D., K. Andersen, J. P. Larsen, A. Lolk, and P. K. Sorensen. 2003. Prevalence and characteristics of dementia in Parkinson's disease. *Arch Neurol* 60:387–92.

Cummings, J. L. 1988. The dementias of Parkinson's disease: Prevalence, characteristics, neurobiology, and comparison with dementia of the Alzheimer's type. *Eur Neurol* 28 Suppl 1:15–23.

Emre, M. 2003. Dementia associated with Parkinson's disease. *Lancet Neurology* 2:229–37.

Mild Cognitive Impairment

Bennett, D. A., J. A. Schneider, J. L. Bienias, D. A. Evans, and R. S. Wilson. 2005. Mild cognitive impairment is related to Alzheimer's disease pathology and cerebral infarctions. *Neurology* 64:834–41.

DeCarli, C., 2003. Mild cognitive impairment: Prevalence, prognosis, etiology, and treatment. *Lancet Neurol* 2:15–21.

Grundman, M., R. C. Petersen, S. H. Ferris, et al. 2004. Mild cognitive impairment can be distinguished from Alzheimer's disease and normal aging for clinical trials. *Arch Neurol* 61:59–66.

Morris, M. C., M. Storandt, J. P. Miller, et al. Mild cognitive impairment represents early-stage Alzheimer's disease. *Arch Neurol* 58:397–405.

Petersen, R. C., G. E. Smith, S. C. Waring, R. J. Ivnik, and E. G. Tangalos. 1999. Mild cognitive impairment: clinical characterization and outcome. *Arch Neurol* 56:303–8.

Petersen, R. C. 2003. *Mild cognitive impairment: Aging to Alzheimer's disease.* New York: Oxford University Press, 1–14.

———. 2004. Mild cognitive impairment as a diagnostic entity. *J Intern Med* 256:183–94.

Petersen, R. C., and J. C. Morris. 2005. Mild cognitive impairment as a clinical entity and treatment target. *Arch Neurol* 62.

Winblad, B., K. Paler, M. Kivipelso, et al. 2004. Mild cognitive impairment: Beyond controversies, towards a consensus—Report of the International Working Group on Mild Cognitive Impairment. *J Intern Med* 256:240–46.

2. Alzheimer's and the Brain

Plaques and Tangles

Bennett, D. A., J. A. Schneider, J. L. Bienias, D. A. Evans, and R. S. Wilson. 2005. Mild cognitive impairment is related to Alzheimer's disease pathology and cerebral infarctions. *Neurology* 64:834–41.

Lopez, O. L., and S. T. DeKosky. 2003. Neuropathology of Alzheimer's disease and mild cognitive impairment. *Rev Neurol* 37:155–63.

Hyman, B. T., and J. Q. Trojanowski. 1997. Consensus recommendations for the postmortem diagnosis of Alzheimer disease from the National Institute on Aging and the Reagan Institute Working Group on diagnostic criteria for the neuropathological assessment of Alzheimer disease. *J Neuropathol Exp Neurol* 56:1095–97.

Mirra, S. S., A. Heyman, D. McKeel, et al. 1991. The Consortium to Establish a Registry for Alzheimer's Disease (CERAD). Part II. Standardization of the neuropathologic assessment of Alzheimer's disease. *Neurology* 41: 479–86.

Braak, H., and E. Braak. 1991. Demonstration of amyloid deposits and neurofibrillary changes in whole brain sections. *Brain Pathol* 1:213–16.

———. 1991b. Neuropathological staging of Alzheimer related changes. *Acta Neuropathologica* 82:239–59.

Synapse and Brain Chemical Losses

Terry, R. D., E. Masliah, and L. A. Hansen. 1999. The neuropathology of Alzheimer disease and the structural basis of its cognitive alterations. In *Alzheimer Disease*, ed. R. D. Terry, R. Katzman, K. L. Bick, and S. Sisodia. Philadelphia: Lippincott, Williams and Wilkins.

Terry, R., E. Masliah, D. Salmon, et al. 1991. Physical basis of cognitive alterations in Alzheimer's disease: Synapse loss iis the major correlate of cognitive impairment. *Ann Neurol* 30:572–80.

Sabbagh, M. N., R. Reid, J. Corey-Bloom, et al. 1998. Correlation of nicotinic binding to neurochemical markers in Alzheimer's disease. *J Neural Transm* 105 (7): 709–717.

Davis, K. L., R. C. Mohs, D. Marin, et al. 1999. Cholinergic markers in elderly patients with early signs of Alzheimer disease. *JAMA* 281:1401–6.

DeKosky, S. T., M. D. Ikonomovic, S. D. Styren, et al. 2002. Upregulation of choline acetyltransferase activity in hippocampus and frontal cortex of elderly subjects with mild cognitive impairment. *Ann Neurol* 51:145–55.

Tiraboschi, P., L. A. Hansen, M. Alford, E. Masliah, L. J. Thal, and J. Corey-Bloom. 2000. The decline in synapses and cholinergic activity is asynchronous in Alzheimer's disease. *Neurology* 55 (9): 1278–83.

Beach, T. G., W. G. Honer, and L. H. Hughes. 1997. Cholinergic fibre loss associated with diffuse plaques in the non-demented elderly: The preclinical stage of Alzheimer's disease? *Acta Neuropathol* (Berl.) 93:146–53.

Beach, T. G., Y. M. Kuo, K. Spiegel, et al. 2000. The cholinergic deficit coincides with Abeta deposition at the earliest histopathologic stages of Alzheimer disease. *J Neuropathol Exp Neurol* 59:308–13.

3. Is Preventing Alzheimer's Disease Really Possible?

Prevalence of Alzheimer's Disease

Ferri, C. P., M. Prince, C. Brayne, et al., Alzheimer's Disease International. 2005. Global prevalence of dementia: A Delphi consensus study. *Lancet* 366 (9503): 2112–17.

Mortimer, J., L. Schuman, L. French. *Epidemiology of dementing illness.* In Mortimer J., L. Schuman, eds. 1981. *The epidemiology of dementia.* Monographs in Epidemiology and Biostatistics. New York: Oxford Univesity Press, 323.

Schuman, L, ed. 1981. *The epidemiology of dementia.* Monographs in Epidemiology and Biostatistics. New York: Oxford University Press, 323.

Evans, D. A., H. H. Funkenstein, M. S. Albert, et al. 1989. Prevalence of Alzheimer's disease in a community population of older persons: Higher than previously reported. *JAMA* 262:2551–56.

Hebert, L. E., P. A. Scherr, J. L. Bienias, D. A. Bennett, and D. A. Evans. 2003. Alzheimer disease in the US population: Prevalence estimates using the 2000 census. *Arch Neurol* 60 (8): 1119–22.

Jonn, A. F. 1990. *The epidemiology of Alzheimer's disease and related disorders.* London and New York: Chapman and Hall. www.alz.org

Foley, D. J., D. B. Brock, and D. J. Lanska. 2003. Trends in dementia mortality from two National Mortality Followback Surveys. *Neurology* 60 (4): 709–11.

Economic Impact of Alzheimer's Disease

Sloane, P. D., S. Zimmerman, C. Suchindran, et al. 2002. The public health impact of Alzheimer's disease, 2000–2050: Potential implication of treatment advances. *Annu Rev Public Health* 23:213–31.

Brookmeyer, R., S. Gray, and C. Kawas. 1998. Projections of Alzheimer's disease in the United States and the public health impact of delaying disease onset. *American Journal of Public Health* 88:1337–42.

Hill, J. W., R. Futterman, S. Duttagupta, V. Mastey, J. R. Lloyd, and H. Fillit. 2002. Alzheimer's disease and related dementias increase costs of comorbidities in managed Medicare. *Neurology* 58 (1): 62–70.

Brest, R. L., and J. W. Hay. 1994. The US economic and social costs of Alzheimer's disease revisited. *American Journal of Public Health* 84:1261–64.

4. Your Alzheimer's IQ: Know Your Risk

Family History

Bachman, D. L., R. C. Green, K. S. Benke, L. A. Cupples, and L. A. Farrer. 2003. Comparison of Alzheimer's disease risk factors in white and African American families. *Neurology* 60:1372–74.

Breitner, J. C. S., J. M. Silverman, R. C. Mohs, and K. L. Davis. 1998. Familial aggregation in Alzheimer's disease: Comparison of risk among relatives of early and late onset cases, and among male and female relatives in successive generations. *Neurology* 38:201–12.

Devi, G., K. Marder, P. W. Schofiels, M. X. Tang, Y. Stern, and R. Mayeux. 1998. Validity of family history for the diagnosis of dementia among siblings of patients with late-onset Alzheimer's disease. *Genetic Epidemiology* 15: 215–23.

Green, R. C., L. A. Cupples, R. Go, et al. 2002. Risk of dementia among white and African American relatives of patients with Alzheimer's disease. *JAMA* 287:329–36.

LaRusse, S., J. S. Roberts, T. M. Marteau, et al. 2005. Genetic susceptibility testing versus family history–based risk assessment: Impact on perceived risk of Alzheimer's disease. *Genet Med* 7:48–53.

Roberts, J. S., A. Cupples, N. R. Relkin, P. J. Whitehouse, and R. C. Green. 2005. Genetic risk assessment for adult children of people with Alzheimer's disease: The risk evaluation and education for Alzheimer's disease (REVEAL) study. *J Geriatr Psychiatry Neurol* 18:250–55.

Mayeux, R., M. Sano, J. Chen , T. Tatemichi, and Yaakov Stern. 1991. Risk of dementia in first-degree relatives of patients with Alzheimer's disease and related disorders. *Archives Neurol* 48:269–73.

Cholesterol and Homocysteine

Burns, M., and K. Duff, K. 2002. Cholesterol in Alzheimer's disease and tauopathy. *Ann N Y Acad Sci* 977:367–75.

Conquer, J. A., M. C. Tierney, J. Zecevic, W. J. Bettger, and R. H. Fisher. 2000. Fatty acid analysis of blood plasma of patients with Alzheimer's disease, other types of dementia, and cognitive impairment. *Lipids* 35:1305–12.

Frears, E. R., D. J. Stephens, E. C. Walters, H. Davies, and B. M. Austen. 1999. The role of cholesterol in the biosynthesis of beta-amyloid. *Neuroreport* 10:1699–1705.

Poirier, J. 2003. Apolipoprotein E and cholesterol metabolism in the pathogenesis treatment of Alzheimer's disease. *Trends Mol Med* 9:94–101.

Refolo, L. M., M. A. Pappolla, B. Malester, et al. 2000. Hypercholesterolemia accelerates Alzheimer's amyloid pathology in a transgenic mouse model. *Neurobiol Dis* 7:321–31.

McIlroy, S. P., K. B. Dynan, J. T. Lawson, C. C. Patterson, and A. P. Passmore. 2002. Moderately elevated plasma homocysteine, methylenetetrahydrofolate reductase genotype, and risk for stroke, vascular dementia, and Alzheimer disease in Northern Ireland. *Stroke* 33:2351–56.

Korczyn, A. D. 2002. Homocysteine, stroke, and dementia. *Stroke* 33:2343–44.

Herrmann, W., and J. P. Knapp. 2002. Hyperhomocysteinemia: A new risk factor for degenerative diseases. *Clin Lab* 48:471–81.

Apolipoprotein E Genotype

Czech, C., H. Forstl, F. Hentschel, et al. 1994. Apolipoprotein E-4 gene dose in clinically diagnosed Alzheimer's disease: Prevalence, plasma, cholesterol levels and cerebrovascular change. *Eur Arch Psychiatry Clin Neurosci* 243: 291–92.

Feskens, E. J., L. M. Havekes, S. Kalmijn, P. de Knijff, L. J. Launer, and D. Kromhout. 1994. Apolipoprotein e4 allele and cognitive decline in elderly men. *BMJ* 309 (6963): 1202–6.

Graff-Radford, N. R., R. C. Green, R. Go, et al. 2002. Association between apolipoprotein E genotype and Alzheimer's disease in African American subjects. *Arch Neurol* 59:594–600.

Henderson, A. S., S. Easteal, A. F. Jorm, et al. 1995. Apolipoprotein E allele epsilon 4, dementia, and cognitive decline in a population sample. *Lancet* 346 (8987): 1387–90.

Green, R. C. 2002. Risk assessment for Alzheimer's disease with genetic susceptibility testing: Has the moment arrived? *Alz Care Quarterly* 3:208–14.

Hurley, A. C., R. Harvey, J. S. Roberts, et al. 2005. Genetic susceptibility for Alzheimer's disease: Why did adult offspring seek testing? *Am J Alz Dis* 20:374–81.

Hyman, B. T., T. Gomez-Isla, M. Briggs, et al. 1996. Apolipoprotein E and cognitive change in an elderly population. *Ann Neurol* 40 (1): 55–66.

Jarvin, G. P., E. M. Wusman, W. A. Kukull, G. D. Schellenberg, C. Ye, and E. B. Larson. 1995. Interactions of apolipoprotein E genotype, total cholesterol level, age, sex in prediction of Alzheimer's disease; A case-control study. *Neurology* 45:1092–96

Roberts, J. S., S. A. LaRusse, H. Katzen, et al. 2003. Reasons for seeking genetic susceptibility testing among first-degree relatives of people with Alzheimer's disease. *Alz Dis Assoc Dis* 17:86–93.

Roberts, J. S., M. Barber, T. M. Brown, et al. 2004. Who seeks genetic susceptibility testing for Alzheimer's disease? Findings from a multi-site, randomized clinical trial. *Genet Med* 6:197–203.

Marteau, T. M., S. Roberts, S. LaRusse, and R. C. Green. 2005. Predictive genetic testing for Alzheimer's disease: Impact upon risk perception. *Risk Analysis* 25:397–404.

Depression

Green, R. C., A. Cupples, A. Kurz, et al. 2003. Depression as a risk factor for Alzheimer's disease: The MIRAGE Study. *Arch Neurol* 60:753–59.

5. Diabetes

Craft, S., and G. S. Watson. 2004. Insulin and neurodegenerative disease: Shared and specific mechanisms. *Lancet Neurol* 3:169–78.

Craft, S. 2006. Insulin resistance syndrome and Alzheimer's disease: Pathophysiologic mechanisms and therapeutic implications. *Alzheimer Dis Assoc Disord* 20:298–301.

Kuusisto, J., K. Koivistom, L. Mykkanen, et al. 1997. Association between features of the insulin resistance syndrome and Alzheimer's disease independently of apolipoprotein E4 phenotype: Cross sectional population based study. *BMJ* 315:1045–49.

Steen, E., B. M. Terry, E. J. Ribera, et al. 2005. Impaired insulin and insulin-like growth factor expression and signaling mechanisms in Alzheimer's disease: Is this type 3 diabetes? *J Alzheimers Dis* 7:63–80.

Yaffe, K., T. Blackwell, R. A. Whitmer, K. Krueger, E. Barrett-Connor. 2006. Glycosylated hemoglobin level and development of mild cognitive impairment or dementia in older women. *J Nutr Health Aging* 10:293–95.

Messier, C. 2003. Diabetes, Alzheimer's disease and apolipoprotein genotype. *Exp Gerontol* 38:941–46.

Peila, R., B. L. Rodriguez, and L. J. Launer. 2002. Type 2 diabetes, APOE gene, and the risk for dementia and related pathologies: The Honolulu-Asia Aging Study. *Diabetes* 51:1256–62.

6. Body Weight and Obesity

Obesity

Gustafson, D., E. Rothenberg, K. Blennow, B. Steen, and I. Skoog. 2003. An 18-year follow-up of overweight and risk of Alzheimer's disease. *Arch Intern Med* 163:1524–28.

Kivipelto, M., T. Ngandu, L. Fratiglioni, et al. 2005. Obesity and vascular risk factors at midlife and the risk of dementia and Alzheimer's disease. *Arch Neurol* 62:1556–60.

Stewart, R., K. Masaki, Q. L. Xue, et al. 2005. A 32-year prospective study of change in body weight and incident dementia: The Honolulu-Asia Aging Study. *Arch Neurol* 62:55–60.

Whitmer, R. A., E. P. Gunderson, E. Barrett-Connor, C. P. Quesenberry Jr., and K. Yaffe. 2005. Obesity in middle age and future risk of dementia: A 27-year longitudinal population-based study. *BMJ* 330:1360.

Metabolic Syndrome

Craft, S. 2006. Insulin resistance syndrome and Alzheimer's disease: Pathophysiologic mechanisms and therapeutic implications. *Alzheimer Dis Assoc Disord* 20:298–301.

Eckel, R. H., S. M. Grundy, and P. Z. Zimmet. 2005. The metabolic syndrome. *Lancet* 365:1415–28.

Razay, G., A. Vreugdenhil, and G. Wilcock. 2007. The metabolic syndrome and Alzheimer's disease. *Arch Neurology* 64:93–96.

Vanhanen, M., K. Koivisto, L. Moilanen, et al. 2006. Association of metabolic syndrome with Alzheimer's disease: A population-based study. *Neurology* 67:843–47.

7. Stroke, Cerebrovascular Disease, and Heart Disease

Cerebrovascular Disease

Desmond, D. W., T. K. Tatemichi, M. Paik, and Y. Stern. 1993. Risk factors for cerebrovascular disease as correlates of cognitive function in a stroke-free cohort. *Arch Neurol* 50:162–66.

Gamaldo, A., A. Moghekar, S. Kilada, S. M. Resnick, A. B. Zonderman, and R. O'Brien. 2006. Effect of a clinical stroke on the risk of dementia in a prospective cohort. *Neurology* 67:1363–69.

Luchsinger, J. A., C. Reitz, L. D. Honig, M. X. Tang, S. Shea, and R. Mayeux. 2005. Aggregation of vascular risk factors and risk of incident Alzheimer's disease. *Neurology* 65:545–51.

Regan, C., C. Katona, J. Walker, J. Hooper, J. Donovan, and G. Livingston. 2006. Relationship of vascular risk to the progression of Alzheimer disease. *Neurology* 67:1357–62.

DeCarli, C. 2003. The role of cerebrovascular disease in dementia. *Neurologist* 9:123–36.

Jellinger, K. A. 2002. Alzheimer's disease and cerebrovascular pathology: an update. *J Neural Transm* 109:813–36.

Pantoni, L., V. Palumbo, and C. Sarti. 2002. Pathological lesions in vascular dementia. *Ann NY Acad Sci* 977:279–91.

Vinters, H. V., W. G. Ellis, C. Zarow, et al. 2000. Neuropathologic substrates of ischemic vascular dementia. *J Neuropathol Exp Neurol* 59:931–45.

Hachinski, V., and D. Munoz. 2000. Vascular factors in cognitive impairment—where are we now? *Ann NY Acad Sci* 903:1–5.

de la Torre, J. C. 2002. Alzheimer's disease as a vascular disorder: Nosological evidence. *Stroke* 33:1152–62.

Erkinjuntti, T. 1999. Cerebrovascular dementia: Pathophysiology, diagnosis, and treatment. *CNS Drugs* 9 (12): 35–48.

Roman, G. 2001. Diagnosis of vascular dementia and Alzheimer's disease. *International Journal of Clinical Practice* 120 (suppl): S9–13.

Roher, A. E., C. Esh, T. A. Kokjohn, et al. 2003. Circle of Willis atherosclerosis is a risk factor for sporadic Alzheimer's disease, arterioscler. *Thromb Vasc Biol* 23:2055-2062.

Kalback, W., C. Esh, E. M. Castano, et al. 2004. Atherosclerosis, vascular amyloidosis and brain hypoperfusion in the pathogenesis of sporadic Alzheimer's disease. *Neurol Res* 26:525–39.

Cardiovascular Disease

Sparks, D. L., J. C. Hunsaker, S. W. Scheff, R. J. Kryscio, J. L. Henson, and W. R. Markesbery. 1990. Cortical senile plaques in coronary artery disease, aging and Alzheimer's disease. *Neurobiol Aging* 11:601–7.

Sparks, D. L. 1997. Coronary artery disease, hyperlipidemia and cholesterol: A link to Alzheimer's disease. *Ann NY Acad Sci* 826:128–46.

Whitmer, R. A., S. Sidney, J. Selby, S. C. Johnston, and K. Yaffe. 2005. Midlife cardiovascular risk factors and risk of dementia in late life. *Neurology* 64:277–81.

Breteler, M. M., J. J. Claus, D. E. Grobbee, and A. Hofman. 1994. Cardiovascular disease distribution of cognitive function in elderly people: The Rotterdam study. *Br Med J* 308:1604–8.

Kivipelto, M., E. L. Helkala, M. P. Laakso, et al. 2001. Midlife vascular risk factors and Alzheimer's disease in later life: Longitudinal, population-based study. *Br Med J* 322:1447–51.

Knopman, D., L. L. Boland, T. Mosley, et al. 2001. Cardiovascular risk factors and cognitive decline in middle-aged adults. *Neurology* 56:42–48.

Hofman, A., A. Ott, M. M. Breteler, et al. 1997. Atherosclerosis, apolipoprotein E, and prevalence of dementia and Alzheimer's disease in the Rotterdam Study. *Lancet* 349:151–54.

Fitzpatrick, A. L., L. H. Kuller, D. G. Ives, et al. 2004. Incidence and prevalence of dementia in the Cardiovascular Health Study. *J Am Geriatr Soc* 52: 195–204.

8. Cognitive Killers

Toxic Exposures

Agronin, M. E. 2006. Dementia due to toxic exposure. *CNS News* 9:36–39.

Albin, R. L. 2000. Basal ganglia neurotoxins. *Neurol Clin* 18:665–80.

Calne, D. B., N. S. Chu, C. C. Huang, et al. 1994. Manganism and idiopathic parkinsonism: Similarities and differences. *Neurology* 44:1583–86.

Hu, H. 2000. Exposure to metal. *Prim Care* 27:983–96.

Peters, H. A., R. L. Levine, C. G. Matthews, et al. 1988. Extrapyramidal and other neurologic manifestations associated with chronic carbon disulfide fumigant exposure. *Arch Neurol* 45:537.

Smoking

Almeida, O. P., G. K. Hulse, D. Lawrence, and L. Flicker. 2002. Smoking as a risk factor for Alzheimer's disease: Contrasting evidence from a systematic review of case-control and cohort studies. *Addiction* 97:15–28.

Merchant, C., M. X. Tang, S. Albert, J. Manly, Y. Stern, and R. Mayeux. 1999. The influence of smoking on the risk of Alzheimer's disease. *Neurology* 52:1408–12.

Ott, A., A. J. Slooter, A. Hofman, et al. 1998. Smoking and risk of dementia and Alzheimer's disease in a population-based cohort study: The Rotterdam Study. *Lancet* 351:1840–43.

Sabbagh, M. N., R. J. Lukas, D. L. Sparks, and R. T. Reid. 2002. The nicotinic acetylcholine receptor, smoking, and Alzheimer's disease *Journal of Alzheimer's Disease* 4 (4): 317–25.

Sabbagh, M. N., S. L. Tyas, S. C. Emery, et al. 2005. Smoking affects the phenotype of Alzheimer's disease. *Neurology* 64 (7) (Apr 12):1301–3.

Depression

Devanand, D. P., M. Sano, M. X. Tang, et al. 1996. Depressed mood and the incidence of Alzheimer's disease in the community elderly. *Arch Gen Psychiatry* 53:175–82.

Green, R. C., A. Cupples, A. Kurz, et al. 2003. Depression as a risk factor for Alzheimer's disease: The MIRAGE Study. *Arch Neurol* 60:753–59.

Head Injury and Boxing

Blennow, K., C. Popa, A. Rasulzada, L. Minthon, A. Wallin, and H. Zetterberg. 2005. There is a strong evidence that professional boxing results in chronic brain damage. The more head punches during a boxer's career, the bigger is the risk. *Lakartidningen* 102 (36) (Sept 5–11): 2468–70, 2472–75.

Szczygielski, J., A. Mautes, W. I. Steudel, P. Falkai, T. A. Bayer, and O. Wirths. 2005. Traumatic brain injury: Cause or risk of Alzheimer's disease? A review of experimental studies. *J Neural Transm* 112 (11) (Nov): 1547–64.

Jellinger, K. A. 2004. Head injury and dementia. *Curr Opin Neurol* 17 (6) (Dec): 719–23.

9. Blood Pressure and Hypertension

Association between Blood Pressure and Dementia

Launer, L. J., G. W. Ross, H. Petrovitch, et al. 2000. Midlife blood pressure and dementia: The Honolulu-Asia aging study. *Neurobiol Aging* 21:49–55.

Fujishima, M., and Tsuchihashi, T. 1999. Hypertension and dementia. *Clin Exp Hypertens* 21:927–35.

Glynn, R. J., L. A. Beckett, L. E. Hebert, M. C. Morris, P. A. Scherr, and D. A. Evans. 1999. Current and remote blood pressure and cognitive decline. *JAMA* 28:438–45.

Hebert, L. E., P. A. Scherr, D. A. Bennett, et al. 2004. Blood pressure and late-life cognitive function change: A biracial longitudinal population study. *Neurology* 62:2021–24.

Kivipelto, M., E. L. Helkala, M. Hallikaien, et al. 2000. Elevated systolic blood pressure and high cholesterol levels at mid-life are risk factors for late-life dementia. *Neurobiol Aging* 21:S174.

Morris, M. C., P. A. Scherr, L. E. Hebert, R. J. Glynn, D. A. Bennett, and D. A. Evans. 2001. Association of incident Alzheimer disease and blood pressure measured from 13 years before to 2 years after diagnosis in a large community study. *Arch Neurol* 58:1640–46.

Morris, M. C., P. A. Scherr, L. E. Hebert, et al. 2002. Association between blood pressure and cognitive function in a biracial community population of older persons. *Neuroepidemiology* 21:123–30.

Prince, M., M. Cullen, and A. Mann. 1994. Risk factor for Alzheimer's disease and dementia: a case-control study based on the MRC elderly hypertension trial. *Neurology* 44:97–104.

Skoog, I., B. Lernfelt, S. Landahl, et al. 1996. 15-year longitudinal study of blood pressure and dementia. *Lancet* 347:1141–45.

Van Dijk, E. J., M. M. Breteler, R. Schmidt, et al. 2004. The association between blood pressure, hypertension, and cerebral white matter lesions cardiovascular determinants of dementia study. *Hypertension* 44:625–30.

Clinical Studies on Effects of Blood Pressure Medications on Dementia

Peila, R., L. R. White, K. Masaki, H. Petrovitch, and L. J. Launer. 2006. Reducing the risk of dementia: Efficacy of long-term treatment of hypertension. *Stroke* 37:1165–70.

Forette, F., M. L. Seux, J. A. Staessen, et al. 1998. Prevention of dementia in randomised double-blind placebo-controlled Systolic Hypertension in Europe (Syst-Eur) trial. *Lancet* 352 (9137): 1347–51.

10. Estrogen and Hormone Replacement Therapy

Scientific Studies on Estrogen and Dementia

Henderson, V. W. 2000. Oestrogens and dementia. *Novartis Found Symp* 230:254–65.

Honjo, H., N. Kikuchi, T. Hosoda, et al. 2001. Alzheimer's disease and estrogen. *J of Steroid Biochemistry and Molecular Biology* 76:227–30.

Li, R., and Y. Shen. 2005. Estrogen and brain: Synthesis, function and disease. *Frontiers in Biosciences* 10:257–67.

Panidis, D. K., Matalliotakis, I. M., Rousso, Dd. H., Kourtis, A. I., Koumantakis, E. E., The role of estrogen replacement therapy in Alzheimer's disease. *Eur J of Obs Gyn Repro Bio* 95:86–91 (2001).

Epidemiological Studies on Estrogen and Dementia

Henderson, V. W., A. Paganini-Hill, C. K. Emanuel, M. E. Dunn, and J. G. Buckwalter. 1994. Estrogen replacement therapy in older women: Comparisons between Alzheimer's disease cases and nondemented control subjects. *Arch Neurol* 51 (9): 896–900.

Kawas, C., S. Resnick, A. Morrison, et al. 1997. A prospective study of estrogen replacement therapy and the risk of developing Alzheimer's disease: The Baltimore Longitudinal Study of Aging. *Neurology* 48 (6): 1517–21.

Zandi, P. P., M. C. Carlson, B. L. Plassman, et al. 2002. Hormone replacement therapy and incidence of Alzheimer's disease in older women: The Cache County Study. *JAMA* 288:2123.

Woods, N. F., E. S. Mitchell, and C. Adams. 2000. Memory functioning among midlife women: Observations from the Seattle Midlife Women's Health Study. *Menopause.* 7 (4) (July–Aug): 257–65.

Clinical Studies on Estrogen, Women's Health, and Dementia

Anderson, G. L., M. Limacher, A. R. Assaf, et al., Women's Health Initiative Steering Committee. 2004. Effects of conjugated equine estrogen in postmenopausal women with hysterectomy: The Women's Health Initiative randomized controlled trial. *JAMA* 291 (14): 1701–12.

Anderson, G. L., H. L. Judd, A. M. Kaunitz, et al., Women's Health Initiative Investigators. 2003. Effects of estrogen plus progestin on gynecologic cancers and associated diagnostic procedures: The Women's Health Initiative randomized trial. *JAMA* 290 (13): 1739–48.

Chlebowski, R. T., S. L. Hendrix, R. D. Langer, et al., Women's Health Initiative Investigators. 2003. Influence of estrogen plus progestin on breast cancer and mammography in healthy postmenopausal women: the Women's Health Initiative Randomized Trial. *JAMA* 289 (24): 3243–53.

Shumaker, S. A, B. A. Reboussin, M. A. Espeland, et al. 1998. Women's Health Initiative Memory Study (WHIMS): A trial of the effect of estrogen therapy in preventing and slowing the progression of dementia. *Control Clin Trials* 19 (6): 604–21.

Shumaker, S. A., C. Legauilt, S. T. Rapp, et al., for the WHIMS Investigators. 2003. Estrogen plus progestin and the incidence of dementia and mild cognitive impairment in postmenopausal women. The Women's Health Initiative Memory Study: a randomized controlled trial. *JAMA* 289 (20): 2651–62.

Mulnard, R.A., C. W. Cotman, C. Kawas, et al. 2000. Estrogen replacement therapy for treatment of mild to moderate Alzheimer disease: A randomized controlled trial. Alzheimer's Disease Cooperative Study. *JAMA* 283 (8): 1007–15.

Henderson, V. W., A. Paganini-Hill, B. L. Miller, et al. 2000. Estrogen for Alzheimer's disease in women: Randomized, double-blind, placebo-controlled trial. *Neurology* 54 (2) (Jan 25): 295–301.

Wang, P. N., S. Q. Liao, R. S. Liu, et al. 2000. Effects of estrogen on cognition, mood, and cerebral blood flow in AD: A controlled study. *Neurology* 54 (11) (Jun 13): 2061–66.

11. Eating Your Way out of Alzheimer's

Saturated Fat

Ervin, R. W., and J. Kennedy-Stephenson. 2005. Dietary intake of fats and fatty acids for the United States population: 1999–2000. Advance Data from Vital and Health Statistics 2004. In *DHHS Publican No. (PHS)* 348, 1240 04–0565.

Kalmijn, S., L. J. Launer, A. Ott, J. C. Witteman, A. Hofman, and M. M. Breteler. 1997. Dietary fat intake and the risk of incident dementia in the Rotterdam Study. *Ann Neurol* 42:776–82.

Morris, M. C., D. A. Evans, J. L. Bienias, et al. 2003. Dietary fats and the risk of incident Alzheimer's disease. *Arch Neurol* 60:194–200.

Morris, M. C., D. A. Evans, J. L. Bienias, C. C. Tangney, and R. S. Wilson. 2004. Dietary fat intake and 6-year cognitive change in an older biracial community population. *Neurology* 62:1573–79.

Fish and Omega-3 Fatty Acids in the Diet

MacLean, C. H., A. M. Issa, S. J. Newberry, et al. Effects of Omega-3 Fatty Acids on Cognitive Function with Aging, Dementia, and Neurological Diseases. Evidence Report/Technology Assessment No. 114 (Prepared by the Southern California Evidence-based Practice Center, under Contract No. 290-02-0003.) AHRQ Publication No. 05-E011-2. Rockville, MD. Agency for Healthcare Research and Quality. February 2005.

Agren, J. J., O. Hannimen, A. Julkunen, et al. 1996. Fish diet, fish oil and docosahexaenoic acid rich oil lower fasting and postprandial plasma lipid levels. *Eur J Clin Nutr* 50:765–71.

Barberger-Gateau, P., L. Letenneur, V. Deschamps, K. Peres, J. F. Dartigues, and S. Renaud. 2002. Fish, meat, and risk of dementia: Cohort study. *BMJ* 325:932–33.

Kalmijn, S., M. P. van Boxtel, M. Ocke, W. M. Verschuren, D. Kromhout, and L. J. Launer. 2004. Dietary intake of fatty acids and fish in relation to cognitive performance at middle age. *Neurology* 62:275–80.

Morris, M. C., D. A. Evans, J. L. Bienias, et al. 2003. Consumption of fish and n-3 fatty acids and risk of incident Alzheimer's disease. *Arch Neurol* 60:940–46.

Morris, M. C., D. A. Evans, C. C. Tangney, J. L. Bienias, and R. S. Wilson. 2005. Fish consumption and cognitive decline with age in a large community study. *Arch Neurol* 12:1849–53.

Benton, D. 1998. Fatty acid intake and cognition in healthy volunteers. In *NIH workshop on omega-3 fatty acids and psychiatric disorders*. Bethesda, MD.

Hashimoto, M., S. Hossain, T. Shimada, et al. 2002. Docosahexaenoic acid provides protection from impairment of learning ability on Alzheimer's disease model rats. *J Neurochem* 81:1084–91.

Hashimoto, M., Y. Tanabe, Y. Fujii, T. Kikuta, H. Shibata, O. Shido. 2005. Chronic administration of docosahexaenoic acid ameliorates the impairment of spatial cognition learning ability in amyloid beta-infused rats. *J Nutr* 135:549–55.

Horrocks, L. A., and A. A. Farooqui. 2004. Docosahexaenoic acid in the diet; its importance in maintenance and restoration of neural membrane function. *Prostaglandins Leukot Essent Fatty Acids* 70:361–72.

Lauritzen, L. 2001. The essentiality of long chain n-3 fatty acids in relation to development and function of brain and retina. *Progress in Lipid Research* 40:1–94.

Lim, G. P., F. Calon, T. Morihara, et al. 2005. A diet enriched with the omega-3 fatty acid docosahexaenoic acid reduces amyloid burden in an aged Alzheimer mouse model. *J Neurosci* 25:3032–40.

McLennan, P., P. Howe, M. Abeywardena, et al. 1996. The cardiovascular protective role of docosahexaenoic acid. *Eur J Pharmacol* 300:83–89.

Mori, T. A., I. B. Puddey, V. Burke, et al. 2000. Effect of omega-3 fatty acids on oxidative stress in humans: GC-MS measurement of urinary F2-isoprostane excretion. *Redox Rep* 5:45–46.

Nelson, G. J., P. C. Schmidt, G. L. Bartolini, D. S. Kelley, and D. Kyle. 1997. The effect of dietary docosahexaenoic acid on plasma lipoproteins and tissue fatty acid composition in humans. *Lipids* 32:1137–46.

Salem, N., Jr., B. Litman, H. Y. Kim, and K. Gawrisch. 2001. Mechanisms of action of docosahexaenoic acid in the nervous system. *Lipids* 36:945–59.

Tully, A. M., H. M. Roche, R. Doyle, et al. 2003. Low serum cholesteryl ester-docosahexaenoic acid levels in Alzheimer's disease: A case-control study. *Br J Nutr* 89:483–89.

Vidgren, H. M., J. J. Agren, U. Schwab, T. Rissanen, O. Hanninen, and M. I. Uusitupa. 1997. Incorporation of n-3 fatty acids into plasma lipid fractions, and erythrocyte membranes and platelets during dietary supplementation with fish, fish oil, and docosahexaenoic acid-rich oil among healthy young men. *Lipids* 32:697–705.

Fruits and Vegetables

Morris, M. C. 2006. Diet and Alzheimer's disease: Meeting the challenges. *J Nutr Health Aging* 10:204.

Morris, M. C., D. A. Evans, C. C. Tangney, J. L. Bienias, and R. S. Wilson. 2006. Associations of vegetable and fruit consumption with age-related cognitive decline. *Neurology* 67:1370–76.

Morris, M. C. 2004. Diet and Alzheimer's disease: what the evidence shows. *Med Gen Med* 6:48.

Oxidation and Antioxidants

Practico, D., C. M. Clark, F. Liun, J. Rokach, V. Y. M. Lee, and J. Q. Trojanowski. 2002. Increase of brain oxidative stress in mild cognitive impairment: A possible predictor of Alzheimer's disease. *Arch Neurol* 59:972–76.

Montine, T. J., J. A. Kaye, K. S. Montine, L. McFarland, J. D. Morrow, and J. F. Quinn. 2001. Cerebrospinal fluid abcta42, tau, and f2-isoprostane concentrations in patients with Alzheimer's disease, other dementias, and in age-matched controls. *Arch Pathol Lab Med* 125:510–12.

Montine, T. J., M. D. Neely, J. F. Quinn, et al. 2002. Lipid peroxidation in aging brain and Alzheimer's disease. *Free Radic Biol Med* 33:620–26.

Montine, K. S., J. F. Quinn, J. Zhang, et al. 2004. Isoprostanes and related products of lipid peroxidation in neurodegenerative diseases. *Chem Phys Lipids* 128:117–24.

Kalmijn, S., E. J. Feskens, L. J. Launer, and D. Kromhout. 1997. Polyunsaturated fatty acids, antioxidants, and cognitive function in very old men. *Am J Epidemiol* 145:33–41.

Montine, T. J., W. R. Markesbery, W. Zackert, S. C. Sanchez, L. J. Roberts II, and J. D. Morrow. 1999. The magnitude of brain lipid peroxidation correlates with the extend of degeneration but not with density of neuritic plaques or neurofibrillary tangles or with APOE genotype in Alzheimer's disease patients. *Am J Pathol* 155:863–68.

Morris, M. C., D. A. Evans, J. L. Bienias, et al. 2002. Dietary intake of antioxidant nutrients and the risk of incident Alzheimer's disease in a biracial community study. *JAMA* 26:3230–37.

Kalmijn, S., E. J. Feskens, L. J. Launer, and D. Kromhout. 1997. Polyunsaturated fatty acids, antioxidants, and cognitive function in very old men. *Am J Epidemiol* 145:33–41.

Laurin, D., K. H. Masaki, D. J. Foley, L. R. White, and L. J. Launer. 2004. Midlife dietary intake of antioxidants and risk of late-life incident dementia: The Honolulu-Asia Aging Study. *Am J Epidemiol* 159:959–67.

Green Tea

Ramassamy, C. 2006. Emerging role of polyphenolic compounds in the treatment of neurodegenerative diseases: A review of their intracellular targets. *Eur J Pharmacol* 545 (1) (Sept 1): 51–64.

Mandel, S., T. Amit, L. Reznichenko, O. Weinreb, and M. B. Youdim. 2006. Green tea catechins as brain-permeable, natural iron chelators-antioxidants for the treatment of neurodegenerative disorders. *Mol Nutr Food Res* 50 (2) (Feb): 229–34.

Rezai-Zadeh, K., D. Shytle, N. Sun, et al. 2005. Green tea epigallocatechin-3-gallate (EGCG) modulates amyloid precursor protein cleavage and reduces cerebral amyloidosis in Alzheimer transgenic mice. *J Neurosci* 25(38) (Sep 21): 8807–14.

Mediteranean Diet

Scarmeas, N., Y. Stern, R. Mayeux, and J. Luchsinger. 2006. Mediterranean Diet, Alzheimer's disease, and Vascular Mediation. *Arch Neurol* 63: epub ahead of print.

Scarmeas, N., Y. Stern, M. S. Tang, R. Mayeux, and J. A. Luchsinger. 2006. Mediterranean diet and risk for Alzheimer's disease. *Ann Neurol* 59:912–21.

12. Red Wine and Other Alcoholic Beverages

Stampler, M. J., J. H. Kang, R. Chen, and F. Grodstein. 2005. Effects of moderate alcohol consumption on cognitive decline in women. *NEJM* 352: 245–53.

Cao, G., and R. L. Prior. 2000. Red wine in moderation: Potential health benefits independent of alcohol. *Nutr Clin Care* 3:76–82.

Tomera, J. F. 1999. Current knowledge of the health benefits and disadvantages of wine consumption. *Trends Food Sci Technol* 10:129–38.

[No authors listed] 2007. Red wine might prevent Alzheimer's disease. Moderate consumption could be a factor in reducing or slowing the incidence of AD. *Health News* 13 (1) (Jan): 7–8.

Sherman, F. T. 2006. The case for alcohol in the primary prevention of dementia: Abstinence may be bad for your health! *Geriatrics* 61 (8) (Aug): 10–12.

Deng, J., D. H. Zhou, J. Li, Y. J. Wang, C.Gao, and M. Chen. 2006. A 2-year follow-up study of alcohol consumption and risk of dementia. *Clin Neurol Neurosurg* 108 (4) (June): 378–83.

Pinder, R. M., and M. Sandler. 2004. Alcohol, wine and mental health: Focus on dementia and stroke. *J Psychopharmacol* 18 (4) (Dec): 449–56.

Letenneur, L. 2004. Risk of dementia and alcohol and wine consumption: A review of recent results. *Biol Res* 37 (2): 189–93.

Luchsinger, J. A., M. X. Tang, M. Siddiqui, S. Shea, and R. Mayeux. 2004. Alcohol intake and risk of dementia. *J Am Geriatr Soc* 52 (4) (Apr): 540–46.

Huang, W., C. Qiu, B. Winblad, and L. Fratiglioni. 2002. Alcohol consumption and incidence of dementia in a community sample aged 75 years and older. *J Clin Epidemiol* 55 (10) (Oct): 959–64.

Tanaka, N., T. Asada, T. Kinoshita, F. Yamashita, and M. Uno. 2002. Alcohol consumption and risk of dementia. *Lancet* 360 (9331) (Aug 10): 491.

13. Managing Your Cholesterol and Lipids

Cholesterol and Alzheimer's

Burns, M., and K. Duff. 2002. Cholesterol in Alzheimer's disease and tauopathy. *Ann N Y Acad Sci* 977:367–75.

Frears, E. R., D. J. Stephens, E. C. Walters, H. Davies, and B. M. Austen. 1999. The role of cholesterol in the biosynthesis of beta-amyloid. *Neuroreport* 10:1699–1705.

Galbete, J. L., T. R. Martin, E. Peressini, P. Modena, R. Bianchi, and G. Forloni. 2003. Cholesterol decreases secretion of the secreted form of amyloid precursor protein by interfering with glycosylation in the protein secretory pathway. *Biochem J* 348:307–13.

Kirsch, C., G. P. Eckert, A. R. Koudinov, and W. E. Muller. 2003. Brain cholesterol, statins and Alzheimer's disease. *Pharmacopsychiatry* 36: 113–19.

Li, G., J. B. Shofer, W. A. Kukull, et al. 2004. Serum cholesterol and risk of Alzheimer's disease: a community-based cohort study. *Neurology* 65: 1045–50.

Miller, L. J., and R. Chacko. The role of cholesterol and statins in Alzheimer's disease. *Ann Pharmacother* 38:92–98.

Notkola, I. L., R. Sulkava, J. Pekkanen, et al. 1998. Serum total cholesterol, apolipoprotein Eepsilon4 allele, and Alzheimer's disease. *Neuroepidemiol* 17:14–20.

Petanceska, S. S., S. DeRose, V. Olm, et al. 2002. Statin therapy for Alzheimer's disease: Will it work? *Neurobiol Dis Neurobiol Dis* 19:155–61.

Refolo, L. M., M. A. Pappolla, B. Malester, et al. 2000. Hypercholesterolemia accelerates Alzheimer's amyloid pathology in a transgenic mouse model. *Neurobiol Dis* 7:321–31.

Reiss, A. B., K. A. Siller, M. M. Rahman, E. S. Chan, J. Ghiso, and M. J. DeLeon. 2004. Cholesterol in neurological disorders of the elderly: Stroke and Alzheimer's disease. *Neurobiol Aging* 25:977–89.

Sparks, D. L., S. W. Scheff, J. C. Hunsaker, H. Liu, T. Landers, and D. R. Gross. 1994. Induction of Alzheimer-like beta-amyloid immunoreactivity in the brains of rabbits with dietary cholesterol. *Exp Neurol* 126:88–94.

Sparks, D. L. 1997. Dietary cholesterol induces Alzheimer-like beta-amyloid immunoreactivity in rabbit brain. *Nutr Metab Cardiovasc Dis* 7:255–66.

———. 1997. Coronary artery disease, hyperlipidemia and cholesterol: A link to Alzheimer's disease. *Ann NY Acad Sci* 826:128–46.

Sparks, D. L., M. N. Sabbagh, J. C. S. Breitner, and J. Hunsaker. 2003. Is cholesterol a culprit in AD? *International Psychogeriatrics* 15 (suppl 1): 153–59.

Statins and Alzheimer's

Fassbender, K., M. Simons, C, Bergmann, et al. 2001. Simvastatin strongly reduces levels of Alzheimer's disease beta-amyloid peptides A-beta 42 and A-beta 40 in vitro and in vivo. *Proc Natl Acad Sci USA* 98:5371–73.

Jick, H., G. L. Zornberg, S. S. Jick, S. Seshadri, and D. A. Drachman. 2000. Statins and the risk of dementia. *Lancet* 356 (9242) (Nov 11): 1627–31.

Morris, M. C., D. A. Evans, C. C. Tangney, et al. 2006. Dietary copper and high saturated and trans fat intakes associated with cognitive decline. *Arch Neurol* 8:1085–88.

Refolo, L. M., M. A. Pappolla, J. LaFrancois, et al. 2001. A cholesterol-lowering drug reduces beta-amyloid pathology in a transgenic mouse model of Alzheimer's disease. *Neurobiol Dis* 5:890–99.

Rockwood, K., S. Kirkland, D. B. Hogan, et al. 2002. Use of lipid-lowering agents, indication bias, and the risk of dementia in community-dwelling elderly people. *Arch Neurol* 59 (2) (Feb): 223–27.

Sparks, D. L., D. J. Connor, D. R. Wasser, J. E. Lopez, and M. N. Sabbagh. 2000. The Alzheimer's Disease Atorvastatin Treatment Trial: Scientific basis and position on the use of HMG-CoA reductase inhibitors (statins) that do or do not cross the blood-brain barrier. In *Advances in drug discovery and drug development for cognitive aging and Alzheimer's disease,* ed. Howard M. Fillit and Alan W. O'Connell, 244–52. New York: Springer Publishing.

Sparks, D. L., D. J. Connor, P. J. Browne, J. E. Lopez, and M. N. Sabbagh. 2002. HMG-CoA reductase inhibitors (statins) in the treatment of Alzheimer's disease; one that crosses the blood-brain barrier. *J Nutr Health Aging* 6:324–31.

Sparks, D. L., D. Connor, J. Lopez, et al. 2004. Benefit of atorvastatin in the treatment of Alzheimer's disease. *Neurobiol Aging* 25:DS24.

Sparks, D. L., S. Petanceska, M. Sabbagh, et al. 2005. Cholesterol, copper and a-beta in controls, MCI, Alzheimer's disease and the Alzheimer's disease Cholesterol-Lowering Treatment trial (ADCLT). *Curr Alz Res* 2:527–39.

Sparks, D. L., M. N. Sabbagh, D. J. Connor, et al. 2005. Atorvastatin therapy lowers circulating cholesterol but not free radical activity in advance of identifiable clinical benefit in the treatment of mild-to-moderate AD. *Curr AD Res* 2:343–53.

———. 2005. Atorvastatin for the treatment of mild-to-moderate Alzheimer's disease preliminary results. *Arch Neurol* 62:753–57.

Sparks, D. L., S. Petanceska, M. Sabbagh, et al. 2005. Cholesterol, copper, and statin therapy in AD. In *Alzheimer's Disease and Related Disorders Annual 5,* ed. S. Gauthier, P. Schelten, and J. Cummings, 89–110, London: Taylor and Francis.

Sparks, D. L., M. Sabbagh, D. Connor, et al. 2006. Statin therapy in Alzheimer's disease. *Acta Neurol Scand* 185:78–86.

Wolozin, B., J. Brown, C. Theisler, and S. Silberman. 2004. The cellular biochemistry of cholesterol and statins: Insights into pathophysiology and therapy of Alzheimer's disease. *CNS Drug Rev* 10:126–46.

Wolozin, B., W. Kellman, P. Ruosseau, G. G. Celesia, G. Siegel. 2000. Decreased prevalence of Alzheimer disease associated with 3-hydroxy-3-methyglutaryl coenzyme A reductase inhibitors. *Arch Neurol* 57 (10) (Oct): 1439–43.

14. Exercising Your Way toward Prevention

Clinical Data for Exercise and Alzheimer's Prevention

Kramer, A. F., S. J. Colcombe, E. McAuley, et al. 2003. Enhancing brain and cognitive function of older adults through fitness training. *J Mol Neurosci* 20 (3): 213–21.

Sturman, M. T., M. C. Morris, C. F. Mendes de Leon, J. L. Bienias, R. S. Wilson, and D. A. Evans. 2005. Physical activity, cognitive activity, and cognitive decline in a biracial community population. *Arch Neurol* 62:1750–54.

Maintain Your Brain, www.alz.org.

[No authors listed] 2006. Defeat dementia with diet and exercise. *Health News* 12 (10): 4.

Lautenschlager, N. T., and O. P. Almeida. 2006. Physical activity and cognition in old age. *Curr Opin Psychiatry* 19 (2): 190–93.

Larson, E. B., L. Wang, J. D. Bowen, et al. 2006. Exercise is associated with reduced risk for incident dementia among persons 65 years of age and older. *Ann Intern Med* 144 (2) (Jan 17): 73–81.

Petrovitch, H., and L. White. 2005. Exercise and cognitive function. *Lancet Neurol* 4 (11) (Nov): 690–91.

Scientific Data for the Protective Effects of Exercise

Nelson, R. 2005. Exercise could prevent cerebral changes associated with AD. *Lancet Neurol* 4 (5) (May): 275.

Wolf, S. A., G. Kronenberg, K. Lehmann, et al. 2006. Cognitive and physical activity differently modulate disease progression in the amyloid precursor protein (APP)-23 model of Alzheimer's disease. *Biol Psychiatry* 60 (12) (Dec 15): 1314–23.

Dishman, R. K., H. R. Berthoud, F. W. Booth, et al. 2006. Neurobiology of exercise. *Obesity* (Silver Spring) 14 (3) (March): 345–56.

Briones, T. L. 2006. Environment, physical activity, and neurogenesis: Implications for prevention and treatment of Alzhemier's disease. *Curr Alzheimer Res* 3 (1) (Feb): 49–54.

Albeck, D. S., K. Sano, G. E. Prewitt, and L. Dalton. 2006. Mild forced treadmill exercise enhances spatial learning in the aged rat. *Behav Brain Res* 168 (2) (Apr 3): 345–48.

15. Staying Sharp with Mental Exercises

Bosma, H., M. P. van Boxtel, R. W. Ponds, P. J. Houx, A. Burdorf, and J. Jolles. 2003. Mental work demands protect against cognitive impairment: MAAS prospective cohort study. *Exp Aging Res* 29 (1) (Jan–March): 33–45.

Verghese, J., R. B. Lipton, M. J. Katz, et al. 2003. Leisure activities and the risk of dementia in the elderly. *N Engl J Med* 348 (25) (June 19): 2508–16.

Wilson, R. S., D. A. Bennett, L. A. Beckett, et al. 1999. Cognitive activity in older persons from a geographically defined population. *J Gerontol B Psychol Sci Soc Sci* 54:155–60.

Wilson, R. S., D. A. Bennett, J. L. Bienias, et al. 2002. Cognitive activity and incident AD in a population based sample of older persons. *Neurology* 59:1910–14.

Wilson, R. S., C. F. Mendes de Leon, L. L. Barnes, et al. 2002. Participation in Cognitively Stimulating Activities and Risk of Incident Alzheimer Disease. *JAMA* 287 (6) (Feb 13): 742–48.

Wilson, R. S., D. A. Bennett, J. L. Bienias, C. F. Mendes de Leon, M. C. Morris, and D. A. Evans. 2003. Cognitive activity and cognitive decline in a biracial community population. *Neurology* 61:812–16.

16. Anti-inflammatories and Alzheimer's

Inflammatory Changes in Alzheimer's Disease

Akiyama, H., S. Barger, S. Barnum, et al. 2000. Inflammation and Alzheimer's Disease. *Neurobiol Aging* 21:383–421.

Rosenberg, P. 2005. Clinical aspects of inflammation in Alzheimer's disease. *International Review of Psychiatry* 17 (6): 503–14.

Hauss-Wegrzyniak, B., P. Dobrzanski, J. D. Stoehr, G. L.Wenk, et al. 1998. Chronic neuroinflammation in rats reproduces components of the neurobiology of Alzheimer's disease. *Brain Res* 780:294–303.

Scientific Studies on Anti-inflammatories in Alzheimer's Disease

Gasparini, L., L. Rusconi, H. Xu, P. del Soldato, E. Ongini, et al. 2004. Modulation of beta-amyloid metabolism by non-steroidal anti-inflammatory drugs in neuronal cell cultures. *J Neurochem* 88:337–48.

Gasparini L., E. Ongini, G. Wenk. 2004. Non-steroidal anti-inflammatory drugs in Alzheimer's disease: old and new mechanisms of action. *J Neurochem* 91:531–536.

Weggen, S., J. L. Eriksen, P. Das, et al. 2001. A subset of NSAIDs lower amyloidogenic Abeta42 independently of cyclooxygenase activity. *Nature* 414 (6860): 212–16.

Lim, G. P., F. Yang, T. Chu, et al. 2000. Ibuprofen suppresses plaque pathology in a mouse model for Alzheimer's disease. *J Neurosci* 20:5709–14.

Van Groen, T., and I. Kadish. 2005. Transgenic AD model mice, effects of potential anti-AD treatments on inflammation and pathology. *Brain Res Rev* 48(2): 370-8.

Population Studies on Anti-inflammatories and Alzheimer's

Etiminan, M., S. Gill, and A. Samii. 2003. Effect of non-steroidal anti inflammatory drugs on risk of Alzheimer's disease: Systematic review and meta-analysis of observational studies. *British Medical Journal* 327:128–32.

Szekeley, C. A., J. E. Thorne, P. P. Zandi, et al. 2004. Non-steroidal anti-inflammatory drugs for the prevention of Alzheimer's disease: a systematic review. *Neuroepidemiology* 23:159–69.

McGeer, P. L., M. Schulzer, and E. G. McGeer. 1996. Arthritis and anti-inflammatory agents as possible protective factors for Alzheimer's disease: a review of 17 epidemiologic studies. *Neurology* 47 (2) (Aug): 425–32.

Intveld, B. A., A. Ruitenberg, A. Hofman, et al. 2001. Nonsteroidal antiinflammatory drugs and the risk of Alzheimer's disease. *N Engl J Med* 345 (21) (Nov 22): 1515–21.

Clinical Trials on Anti-inflammatories and Alzheimer's

Aisen, P. S., K. L. Davis, J. D. Berg, et al. 2000. Randomized controlled trial of prednisone in Alzheimer's disease. Alzheimer's Disease Cooperative Study. *Neurology* 54:588–93.

Aisen, P. S., K. A. Schafer, M. Grundman, et al. 2003. Effects of rofecoxib or naproxen vs placebo on Alzheimer's disease progression: a randomized controlled trial. Alzheimer's Disease Coorperative Study. *JAMA* 289:2819–26.

Aisen, P. S., J. Schmeidler, and G. M. Pasinetti. 2002. Randomized pilot study of nimesulide treatment in Alzheimer's disease. *Neurology* 58 (7): 1050–54.

Reines, S. A., G. A. Block, J. C. Morris, et al. 2004. Rofecoxib Protocol 091 Study Group. Rofecoxib: No effect on Alzheimer's disease in a 1-year, randomized, blinded, controlled study. *Neurology* 62:66–71.

Rogers, J., L. C. Kirby, S. R. Hempelman, et al. 1993. Clinical trial of indomethacin in Alzheimer's disease. *Neurology* 43:1609–11.

Scharf, S., A. Mander, A. Ugoni, F. Vajda, and N. Christophidis. 1999. A double-blind, placebo-controlled trial of diclofenac/misoprostol in Alzheimer's disease. *Neurology* 53:197–201.

Thal, L. J., S. H. Ferris, L. Kirby, et al. 2005. Rofecoxib Protocol 078 study group: A randomized, double-blind, study of rofecoxib in patients with mild cognitive impairment. *Neuropsychopharmacology* 30 (6): 1204–15.

ADAPT Study Group. 2007. No immediate reduction in Alzheimer's disease incidence with naproxen or celecoxib: Results from ADAPT. *Neurology* 68 (May 22): 1–9.

17. Vitamins May Protect

B Vitamins

Morris, M. C., D. A. Evans, J. L. Bienias, et al. 2004. Dietary niacin and the risk of incident Alzheimer's disease and of cognitive decline. *J Neurol Neurosurg Psychiatry* 75:1093–99.

Morris, M. C., D. A. Evans, J. A. Schneider, C. C. Tangney, J. L. Bienias, and N. T. Aggarwal. 2006. Dietary folate and vitamins B-12 and B-6 not associated with incident Alzheimer's disease. *J Alzheimers Dis* 4:435–43.

Morris, M. C., J. A. Schneider, and C. C. Tangney. 2006. Thoughts on B-vitamins and dementia. *J Alzheimers Dis* 9:429–33.

Folic Acid

Luchsinger J. A., M. X. Tang, J. Miller, R. Green, and R. Mayeux. 2007. Relation of higher folate intake to lower risk of Alzheimer disease in the elderly. *Arch Neurol* 64:86–92.

Schneider, J. A., C. C. Tangney, and M. C. Morris. 2006. Folic acid and cognition in older persons. *Expert Opin Drug Saf* 5:511–22.

Morris, M. C., D. A. Evans, J. L. Bienias, et al. 2005. Dietary folate and vitamin B12 intake and cognitive decline among community-dwelling older persons. *Arch Neurol* 62:641–54.

Vitamin C

Morris, M. C., L. A. Beckett, P. A. Scherr, et al. 1998. Vitamin E and vitamin C supplement use and risk of incident Alzheimer's disease. *Alzheimer Dis Assoc Disord* 12:121–26.

Quinn, J., J. Suh, M. M. Moore, J. Kaye, and B. Frei. 2003. Antioxidants in Alzheimer's disease-vitamin C delivery to a demanding brain. *J Alzheimers Dis* 5:309–13.

Zandi, P. P., J. C. Anthony, A. S. Khachaturian, et al., Cache County Study Group. 2004. Reduced risk of Alzheimer disease in users of antioxidant vitamin supplements: The Cache County Study. *Arch Neurol* 61 (1) (Jan): 82–88.

Vitamin E

Montine, T. J., K. S. Montine, E. E. Reich, E. S. Terry, N. A. Porter, and J. D. Morrow. 2003. Antioxidants significantly affect the formation of different classes of isoprostanes and neuroprostanes in rat cerebral synaptosomes. *Biochem Pharmacol* 65:611–17.

Montuschi, P., P. J. Barnes, and L. J., Roberts. 2004. Isoprostanes: Markers and mediators of oxidative stress. *Faseb J* 18:1791–1800.

Morris, M. C., D. A. Evans, J. L. Bienias, et al. 2002. Dietary intake of antioxidant nutrients and the risk of incident Alzheimer's disease in a biracial community study. *JAMA* 26: 3230–37.

Morris, M. C., D. A. Evans, J. L. Bienias, C. C. Tangney, and R. S. Wilson. 2002. Vitamin E and cognitive decline in older persons. *Arch Neurol* 59:1125–32.

Morris, M. C., D. A. Evans, C. C. Tangney, et al. 2005. Relation of the tocopherol forms to incident Alzheimer's disease and to cognitive change. *Am J Clin Nutr* 81:508–14.

Petersen, R. C., R. G. Thomas, M. Grundman, et al. 2005. Vitamin E and donepezil for the treatment of mild-cognitive impairment. *N Engl J Med* 352:2379–88.

Reich, E. E., K. S. Montine, M. D. Gross, et al. 2001. Interactions between apolipoprotein E gene and dietary alpha-tocopherol influence cerebral oxidative damage in aged mice. *J Neurosci* 21:5993–99.

Sano, M., C. Ernesto, R. G. Thomas, et al. 1997. A controlled trial of selegiline, alpha-tocopherol, or both as treatment for Alzheimer's disease. The Alzheimer's disease Cooperative Study. *N Engl J Med* 336:1216–22.

18. Supplements: Real Hope or Empty Promises?

Ginkgo Biloba

Sastre, J., A. Millan, J. Garcia de la Asuncion, et al. 1998. Ginkgo biloba extract (EGb 761) prevents mitochondrial aging by protecting against oxidative stress. *Free Radic Biol Med* 24:298–304.

Ahlemeyer, B., and J. Kriegelstein. 1998. Neuroprotective effects of ginkgo biloba extract. In *Phytomedicines of Europe: Chemistry and biological activity*, ed. L. D. Lawson and R.Bauer, 210–20. Washington, DC: American Chemical Society.

Watanabe, C. M., S. Wolffram, P. Ader, et al. 2001. The in vivo neuromodulatory effects of the herbal medicine gingko biloba. *Proc Natl Acad Sci USA* 98:6577–80.

Kleijnen, J., and P. Knipschild. 1992. Ginkgo biloba for cerebral insufficiency. *Br J Clin Pharmacol* 34:352–58.

Oken, B. S., D. M. Storzbach, and J. A. Kaye. 1998. The efficacy of ginkgo biloba on cognitive function in Alzheimer disease. *Arch Neurol* 55:1409–15.

Hofferberth, B. 1994. The efficacy of EGb 761 in patients with senile dementia of the Alzheimer type, a double-blind, placebo-controlled study on different levels of investigation. *Hum Psychopharmacol* 9:215–22.

Kanowski, S., W. M. Herrmann, K. Stephan, W. Wierich, and R. Horr. 1996. Proof of efficacy of the ginkgo biloba special extract EGb 761 in outpatients suffering from mild to moderate primary degenerative dementia of the Alzheimer type or multi-infarct dementia. *Pharmacopsychiatry* 29:47–56.

Le Bars, P. L., M. M. Katz, N. Berman, T. M. Itil, A. M. Freedman, and A. F. Schatzberg. 1997. A placebo-controlled, double-blind, randomized trial of an extract of ginkgo biloba for dementia. North American EGb Study Group. *JAMA* 278:1327–32.

Wesnes, K., D. Simmons, M. Rook, and P. Simpson. 1987. A double-blind placebo-controlled trial of Tanakan in the treatment of idiopathic cognitive impairment in the elderly. *Hum Psychopharmacol* 2:159–69.

Wettstein, A. 2000. Cholinesterase inhibitors and ginkgo extracts—are they comparable in the treatment of dementia? Comparison of published placebo-controlled efficacy studies of at least six months' duration. *Phytomedicine* 6:393–401.

Ernst, E., and P. H. Pittler. 1999. Ginkgo biloba for dementia. A systematic review of double-blind, placebo-controlled trials. *Clin Drug Invest* 17:301–8.

Birks, J., E. Grimley, and M. Van Dongen. 2002. Ginkgo biloba for cognitive impairment and dementia. *Cochrane Database Syst Rev* 4:CD003120.

van Dongen, M. C., E. van Rossum, A. G. Kessels, H. J. Sielhorst, and P. G. Knipschild. 2000. The efficacy of ginkgo for elderly people with dementia and age-associated memory impairment: new results of a randomized clinical trial. *J Am Geriatr Soc* 48:1183–94.

Weber, W. 2000. Ginkgo not effective for memory loss in elderly. *Lancet* 356:1333.

Solomon, P. R., F. Adams, A. Silver, J. Zimmer, and R. DeVeaux. 2002. Ginkgo for memory enhancement: a randomized controlled trial. *JAMA* 288:835–40.

Mix, J. A., and W. D. Crews Jr. 2002. A double-blind, placebo-controlled, randomized trial of ginkgo biloba extract EGb 761 in a sample of cognitively intact older adults: Neuropsychological findings. *Hum Psychopharmacol* 17:267–77.

Pittler, M. H., and E. Ernst. 2000. Ginkgo biloba extract for the treatment of intermittent claudication: a meta-analysis of randomized trials. *Am J Med* 108:276–81.

Drew, S., and E. Davies. 2001. Effectiveness of ginkgo biloba in treating tinnitus: double blind, placebo controlled trial. *BMJ* 332:73.

Ernst, E., and C. Stevinson. 1999. Ginkgo biloba for tinnitus: A review. *Clin Otolaryngol* 24:164–67.

Gilbert, G. J. 1997. Ginkgo biloba. *Neurology* 48:1137.

Vale, S. 1998. Subarachnoid hemorrhage associated with ginkgo biloba. *Lancet* 352:36.

Murray, M. T., and J. E. Pizzorno. 1998.*Encyclopedia of natural medicine.* 2nd ed. Rocklin, CA: Prima Pub.

Omega-3 Fatty Acids: Docahexanonic Acid

Conquer, J. A., M. C. Tierney, J. Zecevic, W. J. Bettger, and R. H. Fisher. 2000. Fatty acid analysis of blood plasma of patients with Alzheimer's disease, other types of dementia, and cognitive impairment. *Lipids* 35: 1305–12.

Agren, J. J., O. Hannimen, A. Julkunen, et al. 1996. Fish diet, fish oil and docosahexaenoic acid rich oil lower fasting and postprandial plasma lipid levels. *Eur J Clin Nutr* 50:765–71.

Calon, F., G. P. Lim, F. Yang, et al. 2004. Docosahexaenoic acid protects from dendritic pathology in an Alzheimer's disease mouse model. *Neuron* 43:633–45.

Davidson, M. H., K. C. Maki, J. Kalkowski, E. J. Schaefer, S. A. Torri, and K. B. Drennan. 1997. Effects of docosahexaenoic acid on serum lipoproteins in patients with combined hyperlipidemia: A randomized, double-blind, placebo-controlled trial. *J Am Coll Nutr* 16:236–43.

Freund-Levi, Y., M. E. Jonhagen, T. Cederholm, et al. 2006. A randomized double-blind trial with omega-3 fatty acid treatment in mild to moderate Alzheimer's disease. *Arch Neuroly* 63.

Hashimoto, M., S. Hossain, T. Shimada, et al. 2002. Docosahexaenoic acid provides protection from impairment of learning ability on Alzheimer's disease model rats. *J Neurochem* 81:1084–91.

Hashimoto, M., Y. Tanabe, Y. Fujii, T. Kikuta, H. Shibata, and O. Shido. 2005. Chronic administration of docosahexaenoic acid ameliorates the impairment of spatial cognition learning ability in amyloid beta-infused rats. *J Nutr* 135:549–55.

Terano, T., S. Fujishiro, T. Ban, et al. 1999. Docosahexaenoic acid supplementation improves the moderately severe dementia from thrombotic cerebrovascular diseases. *Lipids* 34:S345–346.

Tully, A. M., H. M. Roche, R. Doyle, et al. 2003. Low serum cholesteryl ester-docosahexaenoic acid levels in Alzheimer's disease: a case-control study. *Br J Nutr* 89: 483–89.

Salem, N. Jr., B. Litman, H. Y. Kim, and K. Gawrisch. 2001. Mechanisms of action of docosahexaenoic acid in the nervous system. *Lipids* 36:945–59.

Suzuki, H., Y. Morikawa, and H. Takahashi. 2001. Effect of DHA oil supplementation on intelligence and visual acuity in the elderly. *World Rev Nutr Diet* 88:68–71.

Lim, G. P., F. Calon, T. Morihara, et al. 2005. A diet enriched with the omega-3 fatty acid docosahexaenoic acid reduces amyloid burden in an aged Alzheimer mouse model. *J Neurosci* 25:3032–40.

Marangell, L. B., J. M. Martinez, H. A. Zboyan, B. Kertz, H. F. Kim, and L. J. Puryear. 2003. A double-blind, placebo-controlled study of the omega-3 fatty acid docosahexaenoic acid in the treatment of major depression. *Am J Psychiatry* 160:996–98.

McLennan, P., P. Howe, M. Abeywardena, et al. 1996. The cardiovascular protective role of docosahexaenoic acid. *Eur J Pharmacol* 300:83–89.

Curcumin

Ringman, J. M., S. A. Frautschy, G. M. Cole, D. L. Masterman, and J. L. Cummings. 2005. A potential role of the curry spice curcumin in Alzheimer's disease. *Curr Alz Res* 2:131–36.

Huperzine A

Ashani, Y., J. O. Peggins, and B. P. Doctor. 1992. Mechanism of inhibition of cholinesterases by huperzine. *Biochem Biophys Res Commun* 184:719–26.

Bai, D. L., X. C. Tang, and S. C. He. 2000. Huperzine A, a Potential Therapeutic Agent for Treatment of Alzheimer's disease. *Current Medicinal Chemistry* 7:355–74.

Cheng, D. H., and X. C. Tang. 1998. Comparative studies of huperzine A, E2020, and tacrine on behavior and cholinesterase activities. *Pharmacol biochem behav* 60:377–86.

Wang, Y. E., D. X. Yue, and X. C. Tang. 1986. Anti-cholinesterase activity of huperzine A. *Chung Kuo Yao Li Hsueh Pao* 7:110–13.

Xu, S. S., Z. W. Gao, Z. Weng, et al. 1995. Efficacy of tablet huperzine-A on memory, cognition, and behavior in Alzheimer's disease. *Chung Kuo Yao Li Hsueh Pao* 16:391–95.

Xu, S. S., Z. Y. Cai, Z. W. Qu, et al. 1999. Huperzine-A in capsules and tablets for treating patients with Alzheimer's disease. *Acta Pharmacol Sin* 20: 486–90.

Ye, L., and J. T. Qiad. 1999. Suppressive action produced by beta-amyloid peptide fragment 31–35 on long-term potentiation in rat hippocampus is N-methyl-D-aspartate receptor-independent: It's offset by (-)-huperzine A. *Neurosci Lett* 275:187–90.

Zhang, R. W., X. C. Tang, Y. Y. Han, et al. 1991. Drug evaluation of huperzine A in the treatment of senile memory disorders. *Chung Kuo Yao Li Hsueh Pao* 12:250–52.

Zhu, X. C., and E. Giacobini. 1995. Second generation cholinesterase inhibitors: Effect of (L)-huperzine-A on cortical biogenic amines. *J Neurosci Res* 16:1–4.

Geib, S. J., W. Tuckmantel, and A. P. Kozikowski. 1991. Huperzine A—a potent acetylcholinesterase inhibitor of use in the treatment of Alzheimer's disease. *Acta Crystallogr C* 47:824–27.

Hanin, I., X. C. Tang, G. L. Kindel, and A. P. Kozikowski. 1993. Natural and synthetic Huperzine A: Effect on cholinergic function in vitro and in vivo. *Ann N Y Acad Sci* 695:304–6.

Kozikowski, A. P., and W. Tuckmantel. 1999. Chemistry, Pharmacology, and Clinical Efficacy of the Chinese Nootropic Agent Huperzine A. *Accounts of Chemical Research* 32:641–50.

Tang, X. C., X. C. He, and D. L. Bai. 1999. Huperzine A: A novel acetylcholinesterase inhibitor. *Drugs of the Future* 24:647–63.

Sun, Q., S. Xu, J. Pan, H. Guo, and W. Cao. 1999. Huperzine-A capsules enhance memory and learning performance in 34 pairs of matched adolescent students. *Acta Pharmacol Sin* 20:601–3.

Liu, F. G., Y. S. Fang, Z. X. Gao, J. D. Zuo, and M. L. Sou. 1995. Double-blind control treatment of Huperzine A and placebo in 28 patients with Alzheimer's disease. *Clinical Journal of Pharmacoepidemiology* 4:196.

Ma, Y. X., Y. Zhu, Y. D. Gu, Z. Y. Yu, S. M. Yu, and Y. Z. Ye. 1998. Double-blind trial of huperzine-A (HUP) on cognitive deterioration in 314 cases of benign senescent forgetfulness, vascular dementia, and Alzheimer's disease. *Ann NY Acad Sci* 854:506–7.

Pang, Y. P., and A. P. Kozikowski. 1994. Prediction of the binding sites of huperzine A in acetylcholinesterase by docking studies. *J Comput Aided Mol Des* 8:669–81.

Mazurek, A. 1999. An open-label trial of Huperzine A in the treatment of Alzheimer's disease. *Alternative Therapies* 5:97–98.

Choline, Lecithin, and Phosphatidylserine

Canty, D. J., and S. H. Zeisel. 1994. Lecithin and choline in human health and disease. *Nutr Rev* 52:327–39.

Hanin, I., and G. B. Ansell, eds. 1987. *Lecithin:. Technological, Biological and Therapeutic Aspects.* New York and London: Plenum Press.

Little, A., R. Levy, P. Chuaqui-Kidd, and D. Hand. 1985. A double-blind, placebo-controlled trial of high-dose lecithin in Alzheimer's disease. *J Neur Neurosurg Psych* 48:736–42.

Wurtman, R. J., F. Hefti, and E. Melamed. 1981. Precursor control of neurotransmitter synthesis. *Pharmac Rev* 32:315–35.

Allegro, L., V. Favaretto, and G. Ziiliotto. 1987. Oral phosphatidylserine in elderly patients with cognitive deterioration: An open study. *Clinical Trials Journal* 24 (1): 104–8.

Amaducci, L., and the SMID Group. 1988. Phosphatidylserine in the treatment of Alzheimer's Disease: Results from a multicenter study. *Psychopharmacology Bulletin* 24 (1): 130–34.

Caffarra, P., and V. Santamaria. 1987. The effects of phosphatidylserine in patients with mild cognitive decline: An open trial. *Clinical Trials Journal* 24 (1): 109–14.

Cenacchi, T., T. Bertoldin, C. Farina, M. G. Fiori, G. Crepaldi, and participating investigators. 1993. Cognitive decline in the elderly: A double-blind placebo-controlled multicenter study on efficacy of phosphatidylserine administration. *Aging Clinical Experimental Research* 5 (2): 123–33.

Crook, T. H., J. Tinklenberg, J. Yesavage, W. Petrie, M. G. Nunzi, and D. C. Massari. 1991. Effects of phosphatidylserine in age-associated memory impairment. *Neurology* 41:644–49.

Crook, T., W. Petrie, C. Wells, and D. C. Massari. 1992. Effects of phosphatidylserine in Alzheimer's disease. *Psychopharmacology Bulletin* 28 (1): 61–66.

Delwaide, P. J., A. M. Gyselynck-Mambourg, A. Hurlet, and M. Ylieff. 1986. Double-blind randomized controlled study of phosphatidylserine in senile demented patients. *Acta Neurologica Scandinavica* 73:136–40.

Engel, R. R., W. Satzger, W. Günther, et al. 1992. Double-blind cross-over study of phosphatidylserine vs. placebo in patients with early dementia of the Alzheimer type. *European Neuropsychopharmacology* 2:149–55.

Granata, Q., and J. D. DiMichele. 1987. Phosphatidylserine in elderly patients: An open trial. *Clinical Trials Journal* 24 (1): 99–103.

Heiss, W. D., J. Kessler, R. Mielke, B. Szelies, and K. Herholz. 1994. Long-term effects of phosphatidylserine, pyritinol, and cognitive training in Alzheimer's disease: A neuropsychological, EEG and PET investigation. *Dementia* 5:88–98.

Heiss, W. D., J. Kessler, I. Slansky, R. Mielke, B. Szelies, and K. Herholz. 1993. Activation PET as an instrument to determine therapeutic efficacy in Alzheimer's disease. *Annals of the New York Academy of Sciences* 199 (695): 327–31.

Jorissen, B. L., F. Brouns, M. P. Van Boxtel, et al. 2001. The influence of soy-derived phosphatidylserine on cognition in age-associated memory impairment. *Nutritional Neuroscience* 4 (2): 121–34.

Palmieri, G., R. Palmieri, M. R. Inzoli, et al. 1987. Double-blind controlled trial of phosphatidylserine in patients with senile mental deterioration. *Clinical Trials Journal* 24 (1): 73–83.

Schreiber, S., O. Kampf-Sherf, M. Gorfine, D. Kelly, Y. Oppenheim, and B. Lerner. 2000. An open trial of plant-source derived phosphatidylserine for treatment of age-related cognitive decline. *Israel Journal of Psychiatry and Related Sciences* 37 (4): 302–7.

Sinforiani, E., C. Agostinis, P. Merlo, S. Gualteri, M. Mauri, and A. Mancuso. 1987. Cognitive Decline in Ageing Brain: Therapeutic Approach with Phosphatidylserine. *Clinical Trials Journal* 24 (1): 115–24.

Villardita, C., S. Grioli, G. Salmeri, F. Nicoletti, and G. Pennisi. 1987. Multicentre clinical trial of brain PS in elderly patients with intellectual deterioration. *Clinical Trials Journal*; 24 (1): 84–93.

DHEA and DMAE

Araghiniknan, M., S. Chung, T. Nelson-White, et al. 1996. Antioxidant activity of Dioscorea and dehydroepiandrosterone (DHEA) in older humans. *Life Sciences* 59:147–57.

Baulieu, E. E, and P. Robel. 1998. Dehydroepiandrosterone (DHEA) and dehydroepiandrosterone sulfate (DHEAS) as neuroactive neurosteroids (Commentary). *Proc Natl Acad Sci* 95:4089–91.

Berr, C., S. Lafont, B. Debuire, et al. 1996. Relationships of dehydroepiandrosterone sulfate in the elderly with functional, psychological, and mental status, and short-term mortality: A French community-based study. *Proc Natl Acad Sci* 93:13410–15.

Cardounel, A., W. Regelson, and M. Kalimi. 1999. Deyhydroepiandrosterone protects hippocampal neurons against neurotixin-induced cell death: Mechanism of action. *Proc Soc Exp Biol Med* 222:145–49.

Kimonides, V. G., K. H. Khatibi, C. N. Svendsen, et al. 1998. Dehydrocepiandrosterone (DHEA) and DHEA-sulfate (DHEAS) protect hippocampal neurons against excitatory amino acid-induced neurotoxicity. *Proc Natl Acad Sci* 95:1852–1857.

Kroboth, P. D., F. S. Salek, A. L. Pittenger, et al. 1999. DHEA and DHEA-S: A review. *J Clin Pharmacol* 39:327–48.

Morales, A.J., J. J. Nolan, J. C. Nelson, and S. C. C. Yen. 1994. Effects of replacement dose of dehydroepiandrosterone in men and women of advancing age. *J Clin Endocrinol Metab* 78:1360–67.

Skolnick, A. A. 1996. Scientific verdict still out on DHEA. *J Am Med Assoc* 276:1365–67.

Pfeiffer, C., E.H. Jenney, W. Gallagher, et al. 1957. Stimulant effect of 2-dimethylaminoethanol; possible precursor of brain acetylcholine. *Science* 126 (3274): 610–11.

Cherkin, A., and M. J. Exkardt, 1977. Effects of dimethylaminoethanol upon life-span and behavior of aged Japanese quail. *Journal of Gerontology* 32 (1): 38–45.

Fisman, M., H. Mersky, and E. Helmes. 1981. Double-blind trial of 2-dimethylaminoethanol in Alzheimer's disease. *American Journal of Psychiatry* 138 (7): 970–72.

Zahniser, N. R., D. Chou, and I. Hanin. 1977. Is 2-dimethylaminoethanol (deanol) indeed a precursor of brain acetylcholine? A gas chromatographic evaluation. *Journal of Pharmacology and Experimental Therapeutics* 200 (3): 545–59.

Vinpocetine

Bereczki, D., and I. Fekete. 1999. A systemic review of vinpocetine therapy in acute ischaemic stroke. *Eur J Clin Pharmacol* 55:349–52.

Szakall, S., J. Boros, L. Balkay, et al. 1988. Cerebral effects of a single dose of intravenous vinpocetine in chronic stroke patients: A PET study. *J Neuroimaging* 8:197–204.

Vereczkey, L., G. Czira, J. Tamas, et al. 1979. Pharmacokinetics of vinpocetine in humans. *Arzneimittelforschung* 29:957–60.

Ved, X. C., X. C. He, and D. L. Bai. 1997. Huperzine A, a potential therapeutic agent for dementia, reduces neuronal cell death caused by glutamate. *Neuroreport* 8:963–68.

Hindmarch, I., H. H. Fuchs, and H. Erzigkeith. 1991. Efficacy and tolerance of vinpocetine in ambulant patients suffering from mild to moderate organic psychosyndromes. *Int Clin Psychopharmacol* 6:31–43.

Thal, L. J., D. P. Salmon, B. Lasker, et al. 1989. The safety and lack of efficacy of vinpocetine in Alzheimer's disease. *J Am Geriatr Soc* 37:515–20.

Subhan, Z., and I. Hindmarch. 1985. Psychopharmacological effects of vinpocetine in normal healthy volunteers. *Eur J Clin Pharmacol* 28:567–71.

Lakics, V., M. G. Sebestyen, S. L. Erdo. 1995. Vinopocetine is a highly potent neuroprotectant against veratridine-induced cell death in primary cultures of rat cerebral cortex. *Neurosci Lett* 185:127–30.

Pudleiner, P., and L. Vereczkey. 1993. Study of the absorption of vinpocetine and apovincamic acid. *Eur J Drug Metab Pharmacokinet* 18:317–21.

Acetyl L-Carnitine

Brooks, J. O., J. A. Yesavage, A. Carta, D. Bravi. 1998. Acetyl L-carnitine slows decline in younger patients with Alzheimer's disease: A reanalysis of a double-blind, placebo-controlled study using the trilinear approach. *Int Psychogeriatr* 10:193–203.

Bruno, G., S. Scaccianoce, M. Bonamini, et al. 1995. Acetyl-L-carnitine in Alzheimer's disease: a short-term study on CSF neurotransmitters and neuropeptides. *Alzheimer Dis Assoc Disord* 9:128–31.

Virmani, M. A., R. Biselli, A. Spadone, et al. 1995. Protective actions of L-carnitine and acetyl-L-carnitine on the neurotoxicity evoded by mitochondrial uncoupling or inhibitors. *Pharmacol Res* 32:383–89.

Thal, L. J., A. Carta, W. R. Clarke, et al. 1996. A 1-year multi-center placebo-controlled study of acetyl-L-carnitine in patients with Alzheimer's disease. *Neurology* 47:705–11.

Thal, L. J., M. Calvani, A. Amato, and A. Carta. 2000. A 1-year controlled trial of acetyl-1-carnitine in early-onset AD. *Neurology* 55: 805–10.

Hudson, S., and N. Tabet. Acetyl-l-carnitine for dementia (Cochrane review). *Cochrane Database Syst Rev*: CD003158.

Scorziello, A., O. Meucci, M. Calvani, and G. Schettini. 1997. Acetyl-L-carnitine arginine amide prevents beta 25-35 induced neurotoxicity in cerebellar granule cells. *Neurochem Res* 22:257–65.

Pettegrew, J. W., W. E. Klunk, K. Panchalingam, J. N. Kanfer, and R. J. McClure. 1995. Clinical and neurochemical effects of acetyl-L-carnitine in Alzheimer's disease. *Neurobiol Aging* 16:1–4.

Resveratrol and Quercetin

Marambaud, P., H. Zhao, and P. Davies. 2005. Resveratrol promotes clearance of Alzheimer's disease amyloid-beta peptides. *J Biol Chem* 280 (45) (Nov 11): 37377–82.

Bastianetto, S., W. H. Zheng, and R. Quirion. 2000. Neuroprotective abilities of resveratrol and other red wine constituents against nitric oxide-related toxicity in cultured hippocampal neurons. *Br J Pharmacol* 131 (4) (Oct): 711–20.

Frémont, L. 2000. Biological effects of resveratrol. *Life Sci* 66:663–73.

Frémont, L., L. Belguendouz, and S. Delpal. 1999. Antioxidant activity of resveratrol and alcohol-free wine polyphenols related to LDL oxidation and polyunsaturated fatty acids. *Life Sci* 64:2511–21.

Hung, L. M., J. K. Chen, S. S. Huang, et al. 2000. Cardioprotective effect of resveratrol, a natural antioxidant derived from grapes. *Cardiovascular Res* 47:549–55.

Jang, M., L. Cai, G. O. Udeani, et al. 1997. Cancer chemopreventive activity of resveratrol, a natural product derived from grapes. *Science* 275:218–20.

Jang, M., and J. M. Pezzuto. 1999. Cancer chemopreventive activity of resveratrol. *Drugs Exp Clin Res* 25:65–77.

Stavric, B. 1994. Quercetin in our diet: From potent mutagen to probable anticarcinogen. *Clin Biochem*; 27:245–48.

Heo, H. J., and C. Y. Lee. 2004. Protective effects of quercetin and vitamin C against oxidative stress-induced neurodegeneration. *J Agric Food Chem* 52 (25): 7514–17.

Ono, K., Y. Yoshiike, A. Takashima, K. Hasegawa, H. Naiki, and M. Yamada. 2003. Potent anti-amyloidogenic and fibril-destabilizing effects of polyphenols in vitro: Implications for the prevention and therapeutics of Alzheimer's disease. *J Neurochem* 87 (1) (Oct): 172–81.

19. Get Help: Alzheimer's Is Treatable

Diagnostic Tools

Andreasen, N., C. Hesse, P. Davidson, et al. 1999. Cerebrospinal fluid beta-amyloid (1-42) in Alzheimer's disease: differences between early- and late-onset Alzheimer's disease and stability during the course of disease. *Arch Neurol* 56:673–80.

Sunderland, T., G. Linder, N. Mirza, et al. 2003. Decreased beta-amyloid 1-42 and increased tau levels in cerebrospinal fluid of patients with Alzheimer's disease. *JAMA* 289:2094–2103.

Hock, C., S. Golombowski, F. Muller-Spahn. 1998. Cerebrospinal fluid levels of amyloid precursor protein and amyloid beta-peptide in Alzheimer's disease and major depression—inverse correlation with dementia severity. *Eur Neurol* 39:111–18.

Silverman, D. H. 2004. Brain 18F-FDG PET in the diagnosis of neurodegenerative dementias: comparison with perfusion SPECT and with clinical evaluations lacking nuclear imaging. *J Nucl Med* 45 (4) (Apr): 594–607.

Silverman, D. H., and A. Alavi. 2005. PET imaging in the assessment of normal and impaired cognitive function. *Radiol Clin North Am* 43 (Jan 1): 67–77.

Folstein, M. F., and P. R. McHugh. 1975. Mini-mental state: A practical method for grading the cognitive state of patients for the clinician. *Journal of Psychiatric Research* 12:189–98.

Mohs, R. C., D. Knopman, R. C. Petersen, et al. 1997. Development of cognitive instruments for use in clinical trials of antidementia drugs: Additions to the Alzheimer's disease assessment scale that broaden its scope. *Alzheimer Dis Assoc Disord* 11:S13-S21.

Wilson, B., J. Cockburn, A. Baddeley, and R. Hiorns. 1989. The development and validation of a test battery for detecting and monitoring everyday memory problems. *J Clin Exp Neuropsychol* 11:855–70.

Cummings, J. L., M. Mega, K. Gray, et al. 1994. The Neuropsychiatric Inventory: comprehensive assessment of psychopathology in dementia. *Neurology* 44:2308–14.

Morris, J. C., A. Heyman, R. C. Mohs, et al. 1989. The Consortium to Establish a Registry for Alzheimer's Disease (CERAD). Part I. Clinical and neuropsychological assessment of Alzheimer's disease. *Neurology* 39:1159–65.

Kiernan, R. J., J. Mueller, J. W. Langston, and C. Van Dyke. 1987. The neurobehavioral cognitive status examination: A brief but quantitative approach to cognitive assessment. *Ann Intern Med* 107 (4): 481–85.

Solomon, P. R., A. Hirschoff, B. Kelly, et al. 1988. A 7-minute screening battery highly sensitive to Alzheimer's disease. *Archive of Neurology* 55 (3): 349–55.

Froehlich, T. E., J. T. Robison, and S. K. Inouye. 1988. Screening for dementia in the outpatient setting: the time and change test. *JAGS* 46 (12): 1506–11.

Buschke, H., G. Kuslansky, M. Katz, et al. 1999. Screening for dementia with the memory impairment screen. *Neurology* 52 (2): 231–38.

Schulman, K. I. 2000. Clock drawing: Is it the ideal cognitive screening test? *Int J Geriatric Psychiatry* 15 (6): 548–61.

Borson, S., J. Scanlan, M. Brush, P. Vitialano, and A. Dokmak. 2000. The mini-cog: A cognitive vital sign measure for dementia screening in the multi-lingual elderly. *Int J Geriatr Psychiatry* 15 (11): 1021–27.

Galvin, J. E., C. M. Roe, and K. K. Powlishta. 2005. A brief informant interview to detect dementia. *Neurolog* 65:559–64.

Jorm, A. F. 2004. The Informant Questionnaire on the cognitive decline in the elderly (IQCODE): A review. *Int Psychogeriatr* 16 (3): 275–93.

Solomon, P. R., M. A. Ruiz, and C. M. Murphy. 2003. The Alzheimer's Disease Caregivers Questionnaire: Initial validation of a screening instrument. *Int Psychogeriatr* 15 (suppl 2): 87.

Mundt, J. C., D. M. Freed, and J. H. Griest. 2000. Lay person–based screening for early detection of Alzheimer's disease: Development and validation of an instrument. *J Gerontol B Psychol Sci Soc Sci* 55(3): P163–70.

Galvin, J. E., C. M. Roe, C. Xiong, and J. C. Morris. 2006. Validity and relia-bility of the AD8 informant interview in dementia. *Neurology* 67:1942–48.

Wechsler, D. 1987. *Wechsler Memory Scale—Revised Manual*. San Antonio, TX: Psychological Corporation.

Medications to Treat Alzheimer's

Rogers, S. L., R. S. Doody, R. C. Mohs, and L. T. Friedhoff. 1998. A 24-week, double-blind, placebo-controlled trial of donepezil in patients with Alzheimer's disease. *Neurology* 50:236–45.

Rogers S. L., R. S. Doody, R. C. Mohs, et al. 1998. Donepezil improves cogni-tion and global function in Alzheimer disease. *Arch Intern Med* 50:136–45.

Rogers, S. L., M. R. Farlow, R. S. Doody, et al., for the Donepezil Study Group. 1998. A 24-week, double-blind, placebo-controlled trial of donepezil in patients with Alzheimer's disease. *Neurology* 50:136–45.

Rogers, S. L., and L. T. Friedhoff. 1998. Long-term efficacy and safety of donepezil in the treatment of Alzheimer's disease; an interim analylsis of the results of a US multicentre open label extension study. *Eur Neurop-syschopharmacol* 8:67–75.

Corey-Bloom, J., R. Anand, and J. Veach, for the ENA 713 B352 Study Group. A randomized trial evaluating the efficacy and safey of ENA 713 (rivastig-mine tartrate), a new acetylcholinesterase4 inhibitor, in patients with mild to moderately severe Alzheimer's disease. *Int J Geriatr Psychopharmacol* 1:55–65.

Farlow, M., R. Anand, A. Messina, et al. 2000. A 52-week study of the efficacy of rivastigmine in patients with mild to moderately severe Alzheimer's dis-ease. *Eur Neurrol* 44:236–41.

Doraiswamy, P. M., K. R. Krishnan, R. Anand, et al. 2002. Long-term effects of rivastigmine in moderately severe Alzheimer's disease. Does early initiation of therapy offer sustained benefits? *Prog Neuro Psychophamacol Biol Psy-chiatry* 26:705–12.

Rosler, M., R. Anand, A. Cicin-Stain, et al. 1999. Efficacy and safety of rivastig-mine in patients with Alzheimer's disease: International randomized con-trolled trial. *BMJ* 318:633–38.

Tariot, P. N., P. R. Solomon, J. C. Morris, et al. 2000. A 5-month, randomized, placebo-controlled trial of gatantamine in Alzheimer's disease. *Neurology* 54:2269–76.

Raskind, M. A. E. R. Peskind, T. Wessel, et al. 2000. Galantamine in AD: A 6-month randomized, placebo-controlled trial with a 6-month extension. *Neurology* 54:2261–68.

Knapp, P. J., D. S. Knopman, P. R. Solomon, et al. 1994. A 30-week randomized controlled trial of high-dose tacrine in patients with Alzheimer's disease. *JAMA* 271:985–91.

Lovestone, S., N. Graham. R. Howard. 1997. Guidelines on drug treatments for Alzheimer's disease. *Lancet* 350:232–33.

Disease Modification

Leber, P. 1997. Slowing the progression of Alzheimer's disease methodologic issues. *Alzheilmer Dis Assoc Disord* 11 (supp #5): 510–39.

Sabbagh, M. N., M. R. Farlow, N. R. Relkin, and T. G. Beach. 2006. Do cholinergic therapies have disease-modifying effects in Alzheimer's disease? *Alzheimer's and Dementia* 2 (2): 118–25.

Svensson, A. L., and E. Giacobini. 2003. Cholinesterase inhibitors do more than inhibit cholinesterase. *Cholinesterases and Cholinesterase Inhibitors*, ed. Ezio Giacobini (Institutions Universitaures de Geruatrue de Geneve Thonex-Geneve, Switzerland) 13:227–35.

20. The Future of Alzheimer's Disease

PIB-PET and Future Biomarkers of Disease

Fagan, A. M., M. A. Mintun, R. H. Mach, et al. 2006. Inverse relationship between in vivo amyloid imaging load and CSF A,42 in humans. *Annals of Neurology* 59:512–19.

Klunk, W. E., H. Engler, A. Nordberg, et al. 2004. Imaging brain amyloid in Alzheimer's disease with Pittsburgh compound-B. *Annals of Neurology* 55:306–19.

Lopresti, B.J., W. E. Klunk, C. A. Mathis, et al. 2005. Simplified quantification of Pittsburgh compound-B amyloid imaging PET studies: A comparative analysis. *J. Nuclear Medicine* 46:1959–72.

Mintun, M. A., G. N. Larossa, Y. I. Sheline, et al. 2006. [11C]PIB in a nondemented population: Potential antecedent marker of AD. *Neurology* 67:446–52.

Kaye, J. A., T. Swihart, D. Howieson, et al. 1997. Volume loss of the hippocampus and temporal lobe in healthy elderly persons destined to develop dementia. *Neurology* 48:1297–1304.

Reiman, E. M. 2007. Linking brain imaging and genomics in the study of Alzheimer's disease and aging. *Ann NY Acad Sci* 1097 (Feb): 94–113.

Future Treatments

Clark, C. M., and J. H. T. Karlawish. 2003. Alzheimer disease: Current concepts and emerging diagnostic and therapeutic strategies. *Ann Intern Med* 138:400–10.

Fox, N. C., R. S. Black, S. Gilman, et al. 2005. Effects of Abeta immunization (AN1792) on MRI measures of cerebral volume in Alzheimer disease. *Neurology* 64:1563–72.

Ritchie, C. W., A. I. Bush, A. Mackinnon, et al. 2003. Metalprotein attenuation with iodochlorhydroxyquin (clioquinol) targeting Abeta amyloid deposition and toxicity in Alzheimer's disease: A pilot phase 2 clinical trial. *Arch Neurol* 60:1685–91.

Siemers, E. R., J. A. Kaye, M. R. Farlow, et al. 2004. Effect of LY450139, a functional gamma secretase inhibitor, on plasma and cerebrospinal fluid concentrations of A-beta and cognitive functioning in patients with mild to moderate Alzheimer's disease. *Neurology* 62:A174.

Geerts, H. 2007. Drug evaluation: (R)-flurbiprofen—an enantiomer of flurbiprofen for the treatment of Alzheimer's disease *IDrugs* 10 (2) (Feb): 121–33.

Kennedy, G. J., T. E. Golde, P. N. Tariot, and J. L. Cummings. 2007. Amyloid-based interventions in Alzheimer's disease. *CNS Spectr* 12 (suppl 1) (Jan): 1–14.

Doraiswamy, P. M., and G. L. Xiong. 2006. Pharmacological strategies for the prevention of Alzheimer's disease. *Expert Opin Pharmacother* 7 (1) (Jan): 1–10.

Eriksen, J. L., S. A. Sagi, T. E. Smith, et al. 2003. NSAIDs and enantiomers of flurbiprofen target gamma-secretase and lower Abeta 42 in vivo. *J Clin Invest* 112 (3) (Aug): 440–49.

Solomon, B. 2007. Clinical immunologic approaches for the treatment of Alzheimer's disease. *Expert Opin Investig Drugs* 16 (6) (Jun): 819–28.

Solomon, B. 2007. Intravenous immunoglobulin and Alzheimer's disease immunotherapy. *Curr Opin Mol Ther* 9 (1) (Feb): 79–85.

Aisen, P. S. 2005. The development of anti-amyloid therapy for Alzheimer's disease: From secretase modulators to polymerisation inhibitors. *CNS Drugs* 19 (12): 989–96.

Sabbagh, M. N., D. Galasko, E. Koo, and L. J. Thal. (2000) beta-amyloid and treatment opportunities for Alzheimer's disease. *Journal of Alzheimer's Disease* 2 (3–4): 231–59.

Index